THE HANDBOOK OF
BRIEF THERAPIES

Sara Miller McCune founded SAGE Publishing in 1965 to support the dissemination of usable knowledge and educate a global community. SAGE publishes more than 1000 journals and over 800 new books each year, spanning a wide range of subject areas. Our growing selection of library products includes archives, data, case studies and video. SAGE remains majority owned by our founder and after her lifetime will become owned by a charitable trust that secures the company's continued independence.

Los Angeles | London | New Delhi | Singapore | Washington DC | Melbourne

THE HANDBOOK OF
BRIEF THERAPIES
A PRACTICAL GUIDE

EDITED BY
SARAH PARRY

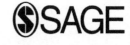

Los Angeles | London | New Delhi
Singapore | Washington DC | Melbourne

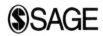

Los Angeles | London | New Delhi
Singapore | Washington DC | Melbourne

SAGE Publications Ltd
1 Oliver's Yard
55 City Road
London EC1Y 1SP

SAGE Publications Inc.
2455 Teller Road
Thousand Oaks, California 91320

SAGE Publications India Pvt Ltd
B 1/I 1 Mohan Cooperative Industrial Area
Mathura Road
New Delhi 110 044

SAGE Publications Asia-Pacific Pte Ltd
3 Church Street
#10-04 Samsung Hub
Singapore 049483

Editor: Susannah Trefgarne
Editorial Assistant: Talulah Hall
Production Editor: Sushant Nailwal
Copyeditor: Sarah Bury
Proofreader: Sharon Cawood
Indexer: Cathryn Pritchard
Marketing Manager: Samantha Glorioso
Cover Design: Sheila Tong
Typeset by: C&M Digitals (P) Ltd, Chennai, India
Printed in the UK

Library of Congress Control Number: 2018955503

British Library Cataloguing in Publication data

A catalogue record for this book is available from
the British Library

ISBN 978-1-5264-3641-2
ISBN 978-1-5264-3642-9 (pbk)

At SAGE we take sustainability seriously. Most of our products are printed in the UK using responsibly
sourced papers and boards. When we print overseas we ensure sustainable papers are used as
measured by the PREPS grading system. We undertake an annual audit to monitor our sustainability.

CONTENTS

CONTENTS

LIST OF FIGURES

LIST OF TABLES

ABOUT THE EDITOR AND AUTHORS

THE EDITOR

Sarah Parry is a Clinical Psychologist within a trauma-informed looked-after children's service and Senior Clinical Lecturer at Manchester Metropolitan University. She is also an enthusiastic amateur furniture upcycler and violin player. Sarah's research interests include therapeutic uses of formulation and the therapeutic utility of compassion for clients and practitioners alike. Sarah and her colleagues also explore how interpersonal trauma can impact aspects of people's lives and how adults and young people develop coping strategies in response to traumatic experiences. Sarah's research has been published in a range of peer-reviewed journals, including the *Journal of Children's Services*, the *Journal of Child Sexual Abuse* and the *Journal of Trauma and Dissociation*.

THE AUTHORS

Panoraia Andriopoulou is a HCPC-registered Clinical and Counselling Psychologist and Senior Lecturer in Psychology at Manchester Metropolitan University. She is fully trained in CBT, Schema Therapy and Systemic Family Therapy and has worked as a practitioner psychologist for more than 12 years, both in private practice and in the public sector, gaining extensive experience in the assessment and treatment of adolescents and adults with anxiety, depressive and personality disorders. Her research interests lie within the areas of clinical/counselling psychology and psychotherapy, psychopathology, psychological wellbeing and the therapeutic properties of close relationships with a special focus on attachment.

Catherine Athanasiadou-Lewis is a Counselling Psychologist and an experienced psychodynamic practitioner and clinical supervisor. She is an HCPC registered practitioner Psychologist, an accredited BABCP CBT practitioner and an Associate Fellow of the British Psychological Society. Catherine is a Senior Lecturer in Counselling Psychology at London Metropolitan University, a Psychology Lead in the NHS, where she practices in the area of substance misuse, and a psychotherapist in Harley Therapy London, where she offers brief and long-term psychodynamic psychotherapy. Catherine conducted her doctoral research on protocol-driven brief therapies where she studied practitioners' experiences of practising Dynamic Interpersonal Therapy as well as Cognitive and Interpersonal Therapies. She has authored a number of papers on psychotherapy and psychopathology and her main research interests include clinical outcomes, psychodynamic psychotherapy, trauma and disorders of the self.

Simone Bol is a Senior Lecturer at Manchester Metropolitan University, with a background in linguistics, social sciences, and speech and language therapy, and is in the final stages of her doctorate in counselling psychology. She is particularly interested in the areas of language and identity and learning and experience.

Gosia Bowling is a lecturer in counselling and psychotherapy at the university of Salford and is also an accredited CBT and EMDR psychotherapist. Gosia works with adults experiencing a wide range of difficulties specialising in trauma and anxiety. She is interested in new therapeutic developments, including third wave CBT and holistic psychotherapies that integrate our understanding of mind and body. Gosia's recent research has investigated the use of CBT and compassion focused therapy for individuals who self harm.

Will Curvis is a Clinical Psychologist at the NHS and a Clinical Tutor on the Doctorate in Clinical Psychology programme at Lancaster University. Clinical and research interests include neuropsychological rehabilitation, pain and long-term health condition management; supporting management and coping around the cognitive, emotional and relational difficulties often seen following brain injury or the development of complex physical health problems. Will is interested in the ongoing development of integrated approaches to psychologically informed healthcare in acute hospital settings.

Venetia Leonidaki is a Clinical Psychologist and an experienced Clinical Supervisor and accredited Dynamic Interpersonal Therapy practitioner. She is also a Visiting Lecturer in Counselling Psychology at London Metropolitan University and a psychotherapist in Harley Therapy, London. Venetia is the co-ordinator of relational therapies in a large NHS service in East London where she acts as Team Leader and offers clinical supervision and training to staff and trainees. She has presented at several conferences and published in academic journals and her main research interests include Dynamic Interpersonal Therapy, qualitative research and psychoanalytic psychotherapy.

Dimitrios Monochristou has been practising as a Counsellor since 2011. He completed his first degree in Psychology at the Aristotle University of Thessaloniki in Greece in 2010. He obtained his Master's degree in Counselling Psychology at Keele University in 2012. Dimitrios has been an accredited member of the British Association for Counselling and Psychotherapy since November 2016 and completed his training as a counselling supervisor with the Macclesfield Counselling and Training Centre in April 2017. Over the last six years he has worked in the community sector, in an NHS IAPT service and in a psychiatric ward at the Oldham and Tameside Burroughs of Greater Manchester. Currently, Dimitrios works as a student counsellor at Manchester Metropolitan University and maintains a small counselling practice in collaboration with fellow counsellors in the Manchester city centre.

Neil Murphy currently leads a postgraduate programme in Cognitive Behavioural Psychotherapy at the University of Salford and has extensive experience related to cognitive, behavioural and family therapy. Much of his current research is related to investigating how various forms of media influence decisions made by practitioners in clinical practice. An important driver for him is to enable people at all levels of training to be able to implement cognitively orientated interventions and to appreciate the impact of how internal and external factors that are outside the control of the individual can influence the practice engaged in.

Jorge E. Palacios is a postdoctoral Clinical Researcher at SilverCloud Health and is Research Fellow at Trinity College Dublin. He recently completed a PhD in Psychological Medicine at King's College London. His thesis focused on the longitudinal symptomatology of depression and anxiety in coronary heart disease. Recent work on the trajectories of symptoms of distress earned him the Young Investigator of the Year Award from the European Association of Psychosomatic Medicine and Elsevier. His main research interests include digital interventions and mobile technology for mental health, and the comorbidity between mental and physical illness.

Derek Richards is the Chief Science Officer at SilverCloud. Derek leads the global research initiatives that impact the development of the SilverCloud solutions. Together with Dr Ladislav Timulak, he is co-director of the E-mental health research group in the School of Psychology, Trinity College Dublin. He is very interested in the development, implementation and research of technology-delivered interventions for mental health. He has presented and published nationally and internationally in this area. www.derekrichards.ie.

Laura Richardson is an HCPC registered art therapist from Sheffield (UK) with 29 years practice. She holds an MA in Art Psychotherapy Practice and Research from the University of Sheffield and Leeds Metropolitan University, a degree in fine art, and a diploma in Continuing Professional and Managerial Development from Sheffield Hallam University. She has worked across the full age range; in the voluntary sector with children and families, in the social services mental health day service, and in NHS adult mental health acute, day hospital, community mental health, and residential dementia care settings. Laura's roles have included being Professional Lead 100 for Arts Therapies and Arts Lead for Sheffield Health and Social Care NHS Foundation Trust, and she has contributed to the Trust's King's Fund- inspired projects to "enhance the healing environment". Now retired, Laura currently provides art therapy supervision, and occasional lecturing for Leeds Beckett University's Art Therapy Northern Programme MA course.

Katy Roe is a Clinical Psychologist who has worked in the NHS for 15 years and had her own private practice for eight years, carrying out clinical work, teaching, training, consultation and supervision. Katy became interested in acceptance and mindfulness based approaches during her MSc at Bangor University in 2001. After qualifying from Liverpool University with a doctorate in 2006, her work has been predominantly in the field of Severe and Enduring Adult Mental Health in a community setting. Katy has a keen interest in organisational wellbeing and preventative mental health work and she is currently working on a collaborative Arts and Science project which is intended to promote emotional learning aimed at primary school settings.

Angel Enrique Roig currently works as a postdoctoral Clinical Researcher at SilverCloud Health and Research Fellow at Trinity College Dublin. He has developed and researched the efficacy of clinical interventions, face-to-face and internet-delivered, for different conditions, such as anxiety, depression and eating disorders. He has completed postgraduate studies in the treatment of eating disorders and has expertise in mindfulness and its applications in clinical practice.

Clive Turpin is a CAT Psychotherapist and supervisor working in a psychotherapy service in North Manchester (accredited and registered with ACAT and UKCP). He has extensive experience of working with self-harm, initially as a nurse therapist on a research project which evolved into a self-harm team offering PIT, based in Central Manchester. Clive has also contributed to other research papers with the Centre for Suicide Prevention and consulted on and supervised for a research project (WORSHIP Study) focusing on providing therapy for women prisoners who have self-harmed. He holds a particular interest in using CAT and PIT in brief formats to improve relational understanding.

Hannah Wilson, DClinPsy, is a Clinical Psychologist working in both the public and private sectors within the North West of England. Her interest in Compassion-Focused Therapy (CFT) started during her clinical psychology training, and she has continued to train in this model and develop her skills ever since. Hannah is currently enjoying adapting her CFT skills for different ages and presentations. She is also on an ever-developing journey of employing these strategies and techniques within her own life and to support her own wellbeing.

ACKNOWLEDGEMENTS

Sincere thanks to James Thomas Yeomans and Lisa Ann Sproson of Manchester Metropolitan University for their research assistance towards this Handbook.

INTRODUCTION

Acting as a therapist can be many things: incredibly rewarding, challenging, inspiring, captivating and creative. However, it can also feel like literally acting without a script, without direction or the opportunity for an edit. In short, talking therapy is live, dynamic and can be demanding for both client and therapist. The role of therapeutic training is often not to provide a series of scripts or structures to choose from, but to cultivate a way of thinking so that the therapist can work creatively and responsively with the client's story, without seeing the script or perhaps meeting the other characters. For that reason, no amount of reading alone can train a therapeutic mind. To become an active agent of change in a meaningful therapeutic alliance requires a great deal of skills practice and reflection on action (reflexive practice). However, the specific goal of *The Handbook of Brief Therapies* is to offer a summary of frequently employed brief modalities, with their unique and shared features, for practitioners at all stages of training and practice. Each chapter aims to demystify a core therapeutic framework that can be delivered in 24 sessions or less. Brief interventions are attractive for clients for a range of reasons, including their focus on tackling a particular difficulty, time requirements, access, financial cost, and their structured style.

Within this *Handbook of Brief Therapies*, each contributor guides the reader through a modality for which they hold a particular passion and interest, discussing the key techniques and practices inherent to that model, and concluding with stories from practice to further guide the reader in the implementation of that model. I conclude the book with a brief introduction to integrative approaches and consider how therapists can draw on different models for a range of desired outcomes. Before that, however, let us consider some key components of brief interventions in practice.

THE THERAPEUTIC RELATIONSHIP

There are many entire books dedicated to exploring the power and complexities of the therapeutic relationship (also called the 'therapeutic alliance' or 'working alliance'), including a particularly good one by Stephen Paul and Divine Charura entitled *An Introduction to the Therapeutic Relationship in Counselling and Psychotherapy*, first published in 2014. Each chapter of this book will consider the development and nature of the therapeutic relationship in a manner consistent with the particular brief intervention presented.

Short-term therapeutic work naturally means the therapist and client typically have fewer sessions together than in longer-term therapy. Therefore, establishing a positive therapeutic relationship from the onset is particularly important. The key messages we need to bear in mind during any therapeutic encounter can be briefly summarised as follows:

- A positive therapeutic relationship is the essential ingredient for positive treatment engagement, outcomes, and overall efficacy of any therapeutic modality (Norcross & Wampold, 2011; Kelly, Greene, & Bergman, 2016).
- Considering the role of Bowlby's attachment theory (1969/1982) for the therapeutic relationship can help us understand how adult attachment styles (Smith, Msetfi, & Golding, 2010), our biosocial need for connection (Fishbane, 2007), and establishing a secure base of support (Berry & Danquah, 2016) can all nurture a positive alliance.
- Across the therapeutic community and literature base, the components illustrated in Figure I.1 are generally regarded as the pillars required to build a safe space within which a meaningful, resonant and dynamic therapeutic alliance can flourish.

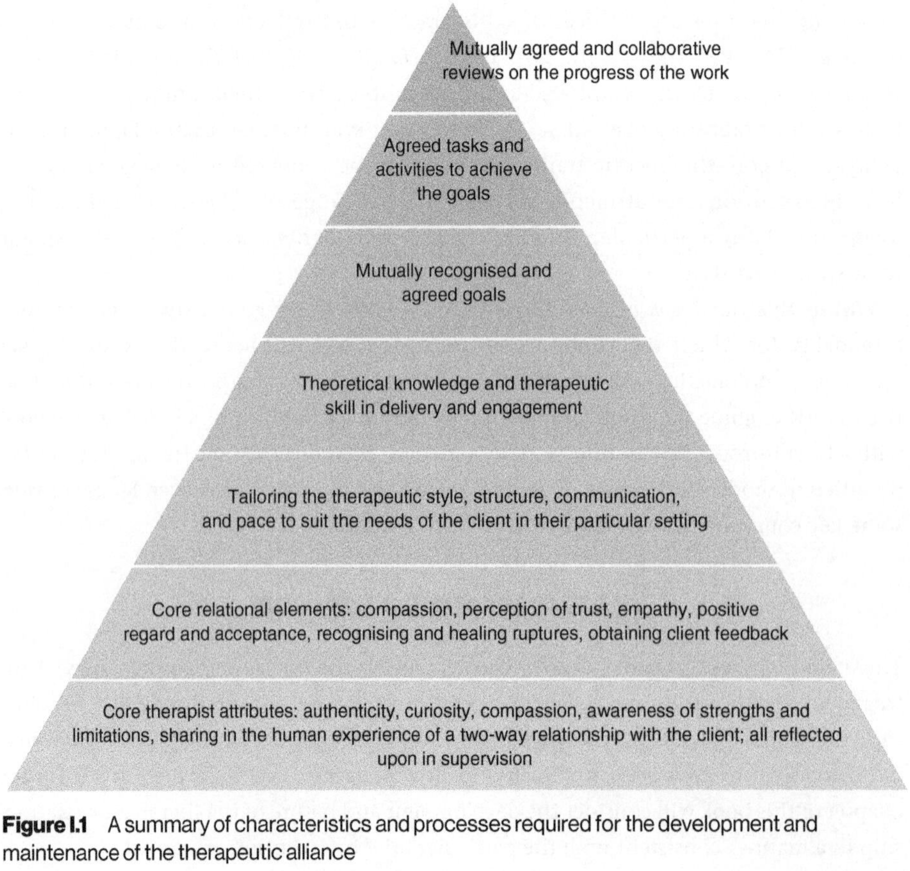

Mutually agreed and collaborative reviews on the progress of the work

Agreed tasks and activities to achieve the goals

Mutually recognised and agreed goals

Theoretical knowledge and therapeutic skill in delivery and engagement

Tailoring the therapeutic style, structure, communication, and pace to suit the needs of the client in their particular setting

Core relational elements: compassion, perception of trust, empathy, positive regard and acceptance, recognising and healing ruptures, obtaining client feedback

Core therapist attributes: authenticity, curiosity, compassion, awareness of strengths and limitations, sharing in the human experience of a two-way relationship with the client; all reflected upon in supervision

Figure I.1 A summary of characteristics and processes required for the development and maintenance of the therapeutic alliance

A recent review and position paper proposed five factors across modalities that were likely to result in positive therapeutic change:

1. The ability of the therapist to inspire hope and to provide an alternative and more plausible view of the self and the world;
2. the ability to give patients a corrective emotional experience that helps them to remedy the traumatic influence of his previous life experiences;
3. the therapeutic alliance;
4. positive change expectations;
5. and beneficial therapist qualities, such as attention, empathy and positive regard (Zarbo, Tasca, Cattafi, & Compare, 2016, p. 2022) (see also Stricker & Gold, 2001; Feixas & Botella, 2004; Norcross & Goldfried, 2005; Constantino et al., 2011; Horvath et al., 2011)

FORMULATION

Across mental health professions, formulation is concurrently known as 'clinical formulation', 'case formulation', the 'cornerstone of therapy', 'solution finding', 'problem formulation' or simply 'meaning making'. Whatever your preferred term, formulation is often the therapist's North Star in terms of making sense of where the therapeutic process is up to, understanding influences upon movement, and what the direction of travel could be with our clients. Personally, I haven't found a better resource for understanding formulation than Lucy Johnstone and Rudi Dallos's *Formulation in Psychology and Psychotherapy: Making Sense of People's Problems* (2013) – a must-read in formulation education. Although formulation is employed implicitly and explicitly in various forms across therapeutic modalities, as the chapters illustrate, formulation's central purpose is to consider how the difficulties a person is experiencing operate in their intrapersonal, social, cultural, environmental and practical milieu, drawing on psychological theory.

The shared understanding of personal experience between client and therapist is a developmental process that occurs and reoccurs at various stages of the therapeutic process, even within brief interventions. The therapist then uses their theoretical knowledge to interpret the client's needs, strengths and difficulties, leading to the co-production of an intervention strategy that should be suitable for the client at that time. Importantly, when undertaken correctly and sensitively, the process of formulation can be incredibly therapeutic, perhaps particularly for people who have felt as though their emotional distress has been overly medicalised into an illness or pathologised into something they have little control over. Delving into the human experience can be a difficult journey, although it can also empower people to understand the causes of their distress and provide new platforms and an opportunity for understanding, intervention, support and hope for healing. Many formulation templates that cross modalities are freely available online, which can be very helpful for practitioners as they become more familiar with the process.

Additionally, the following questions can provide a useful framework when beginning the formulation process with a client in a brief intervention setting:

1. What/who has brought the client to see you?
2. What is the main difficulty the client is trying to address?
3. What coping strategies are they already using that are helpful or unhelpful?
4. What resources does the client have available to them to address the difficulty (personal resilience and agency, social support, financial stability, etc.)?
5. What resource areas might need to be addressed in order to empower the client on a practical basis? Although therapy can be a helpful platform for exploring one's options and making healthy choices, no amount of CBT will help a mother feel less anxious about feeding her children if she just doesn't have the money for food. Similarly, Motivational Interviewing will not encourage an elderly person to put their heating on if there are no coins left for the meter.
6. Once collaboratively developed, how will the formulation shape the direction and travel of therapy? What will need to happen outside the therapy room to make the process worthwhile?
7. Will the formulation be explicitly reviewed at the end of every session, every four weeks, or updated as and when necessary? Explaining these processes explicitly can be containing for the client and invite ownership of the process from the beginning.
8. Does there need to be an additional formulation with further systemic factors included for use in supervision (e.g. considering service structures, resources, therapist–client relational factors)?

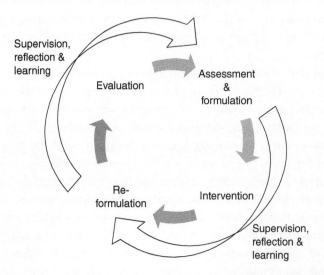

Figure I.2 The process of formulation and reformulation, supported through reflexive practice and supervision

LANGUAGE AND SHARED EXPERIENCE

Throughout this book, you will notice some caution around diagnostic terminology and a recognition that many forms of distress share similar features. The chapters within this book consider how their brief therapeutic approach can be utilised effectively for people with common psychological difficulties, such as feeling anxious or low in mood, which often transcend across a wide variety of diagnostic labels and emotional experiences. Over recent years, critical considerations around the value and even validity of some diagnoses (e.g. personality disorders, schizophrenia) and conceptualisations of traditionally perceived mental health difficulties (e.g. hearing voices) have been vigorously debated across advocacy and professional groups. Critics of the dominant biomedical model of illness state that 'social and economic determinants of mental health demand public health and population-based strategies' for communities (Thangadurai & Jacob, 2014, p. 351), rather than deficit-orientated individualised treatment packages. Others propose that when it comes to understanding mental health in Western societies, science has been replaced by 'social control, political expediency, and professional imperialism' (Sanders, 2015, p. 32).

That said, some people find the diagnostic framework validating, containing and recognising of their difficulties. Additionally, having a diagnosis can, in some cases, open doors to treatment in some healthcare and education settings. Ultimately, there is no easy answer or quick resolution to this debate as it rumbles on. However, we as practitioners need to be mindful that this debate continues and that the biomedical understanding of mental health that prevails in the Western world may not suit all of our clients, meaning that this is another systemic factor we need to build into our formulations and meaning-making processes.

Finally, it is essential that we as practitioners don't fall into the trap of thinking we are immune from emotional distress just because of our day job. In fact, there is growing evidence indicating that people working with the distress and trauma of others are more likely to need emotional support at times (Nimmo & Huggard, 2013; Halevi & Idisis, 2017; Parry, 2017). In terms of keeping ourselves safe at work, my colleagues and I recently found the following was essential for people across sectors working in a therapeutic capacity (Parry, 2017, p. 161):

1. A sense of purpose and belonging – we need to believe in what we are doing and know what we do is seen, witnessed and recognised.
2. A safe and supportive space with colleagues or a supervisor for reflectively processing distressing events and information.
3. Feeling valued and wanted – 'off days' are difficult when your job requires emotional labour as standard, so having an emotional safe-base at work goes a long way!
4. Self-kindness and acceptance – we are not super-human and need to recognise *good enough* sometimes, asking for help when we need it.

BEFORE DIVING IN...

Each chapter of the book follows a similar format to facilitate comparison and reference across chapters. Each chapter begins with a quick introduction to the model and its heritage (summarised in Table I.1), before exploring the theoretical evidence base. A short critical evaluation of each model is also presented as no model (or therapist) is without limitations and shortfalls. From there, the contributing authors discuss a practical 'how to' guide to implementing the techniques and approaches characteristic of that model, consolidated through anonymised case examples from practice. Throughout, top tips, definitions and discussion questions should develop learning and facilitate reflection. A series of references and recommended further reading resources are offered to signpost readers to other materials of use and interest. Enjoy!

Table I.1 Theoretical underpinnings of the modalities presented in *The Handbook of Brief Therapies*

Modality/heritage	Humanistic	Psychodynamic	Evolutionary	Cognitive/ behavioural
Psychoeducation				
Time-Limited Person-Centred Therapy				
Motivational Interviewing				
Solution-Focused Brief Therapy				
Short-Term Family Therapy				
Brief Cognitive Behavioural Therapy				
Internet-delivered Cognitive Behavioural Therapy				
Brief Compassionate Mind Training				
Short Acceptance and Commitment Therapy				
Brief Dynamic Interpersonal Therapy				
Cognitive Analytic Therapy				
Psychodynamic Interpersonal Therapy				
Brief Interventions Using Artistic Expression				
Brief Interventions in Hospital Settings				

REFERENCES

Barber, J.P. (1996). Comprehensive handbook of psychotherapy integration: Edited by G. Stricker & J.R. Gold. New-York: Plenum Press, 1993. 561 pp. *Clinical Psychology Review, 16*(1), 76–78.

Berry, K. & Danquah, A. (2016). Attachment-informed therapy for adults: Towards a unifying perspective on practice. *Psychology and Psychotherapy: Theory, Research and Practice, 89*(1), 15–32.

Bowlby, J. (1969/1982). *Attachment and loss: Vol. 1. Attachment*. New York: Basic Books.

Feixas, G. & Botella, L. (2004). Psychotherapy integration: Reflections and contributions from a constructivist epistemology. *Journal of Psychotherapy Integration, 14*(2), 192–222.

Fishbane, M.D. (2007). Wired to connect: Neuroscience, relationships, and therapy. *Family Process, 46*(3), 395–412.

Halevi, E. & Idisis, Y. (2017). Who helps the helper? Differentiation of self as an indicator for resisting vicarious traumatization. *Psychological Trauma: Theory, Research, Practice, and Policy*, doi: 10.1037/tra0000318.

Johnstone, L. & Dallos, R. (2013). *Formulation in psychology and psychotherapy: Making sense of people's problems*. London: Routledge.

Kelly, J.F., Greene, M.C. & Bergman, B.G. (2016). Recovery benefits of the 'therapeutic alliance' among 12-step mutual-help organization attendees and their sponsors. *Drug and Alcohol Dependence, 162*, 64–71.

Nimmo, A. & Huggard, P. (2013). A systematic review of the measurement of compassion fatigue, vicarious trauma, and secondary traumatic stress in physicians. *Australasian Journal of Disaster and Trauma Studies, 1*, 37.

Norcross, J.C. & Goldfried, M.R. (2005). *Handbook of psychotherapy integration* (2nd ed.). Oxford: Oxford University Press.

Norcross, J.C. & Wampold, B.E. (2011). What works for whom: Tailoring psychotherapy to the person. *Journal of Clinical Psychology, 67*(2), 127–132.

Parry, S. (2017). *Effective self-care and resilience in clinical practice: Dealing with stress, compassion fatigue and burnout*. London & Philadelphia, PA: Jessica Kingsley.

Paul, S. & Charura, D. (2014). *An introduction to the therapeutic relationship in counselling and psychotherapy*. London: Sage.

Sanders, P. (2015). Why person-centred therapists must reject the medicalisation of distress. *Self & Society, 34*(3), 32–39. doi: 10.1080/03060497.2006.11083918.

Smith, A.E.M., Msetfi, R.M. & Golding, L. (2010). Client self rated adult attachment patterns and the therapeutic alliance: A systematic review. *Clinical Psychology Review, 30*(3), 326–337.

Thangadurai, P., & Jacob, K.S. (2014). Medicalizing distress, ignoring public health strategies. *Indian Journal of Psychological Medicine, 36*(4), 351–354.

Zarbo, C., Tasca, G.A., Cattafi, F. & Compare, A. (2016). Integrative psychotherapy works. *Frontiers in Psychology, 6*, doi:10.3389/fpsyg.2015.02021.

PART I
CORE APPROACHES

1

BRIEF COGNITIVE BEHAVIOURAL THERAPY

NEIL MURPHY AND GOSIA BOWLING

INTRODUCTION

Brief Cognitive Behaviour Therapy (BCBT) evolved around 20 years ago from traditional CBT as an evidenced-based and effective short-term treatment option for a range of difficulties.

This chapter aims to:

- discuss the distinct differences of BCBT compared to traditional CBT
- explore both the strengths and limitations of BCBT
- discuss the evidence base for the use of BCBT
- highlight the use of BCBT in practice with an emphasis on its structure and design.

--------- KEY TERMS ---------

Cognitive Behavioural Therapy CBT is commonly described as a 'talking therapy' but is an active and directive form of therapy that acknowledges that an individual's environment, thoughts, feelings, actions and physical reactions are interlinked and changes to one can impact on other parts.

Brief Cognitive Behaviour Therapy BCBT is a compressed or short-term, problem-focused and goal-directed therapy that adopts similar approaches to CBT but in a more time-constrained and active manner for clients with a limited problem profile.

BACKGROUND

BCBT is based on the underpinning theory and application of CBT approaches, which are applicable for a range of people experiencing emotional, physical and social difficulties. BCBT works with cognitions and the interpretations of such cognitions in relation to how the person feels and behaves. It challenges what might be seen as 'maladaptive cognitions' and typically focuses on the identification of automatic thoughts and potential 'thought distortions', especially in early sessions.

Although being cognitive in nature, BCBT and CBT do share specific symptom-reduction principles that are inherent in most medical models. Where BCBT and CBT veer away from this model is in the active participation of the person experiencing the problem and the collaborative nature of the work between client and therapist. More specifically, Bond and Dryden (2008) argued that BCBT should be conducted in fewer than 10 sessions as compared to traditional CBT, which commonly lasts between 10 and 20 sessions. Briefer formats of therapy than the range of 10 to 20 sessions have become commonplace in healthcare practice. The impetus for the move towards a more compressed approach in the UK probably lay with the implementation of Improving Access to Psychological Therapies (IAPT) following the Layard Report in the UK in 2006 (Layard et al., 2006). At this point in time, CBT practice branched out from being the domain of psychologists working in consulting rooms to being utilised by a range of therapists from various backgrounds (nurses, counsellors, social workers, to name a few) in multiple settings.

There is some debate relating to what differentiates BCBT from CBT, which is by nature a very structured, short-term compressed approach. Curwen, Palmer and Ruddell's abridged description of 'a series of sessions of brief cognitive behaviour therapy that uses time flexibly and focusses on client goals using a framework of cognitive conceptualisation' (2018, p. 3) is one we advocate. An important message is that IAPT work and BCBT are not necessarily the same therapy. Although IAPT is not defined as a brief therapy provider, many low-intensity IAPT provisions are delivered in fewer than 12 sessions. Much low-intensity IAPT work involves the use of brief interventions, which can be delivered in person, or through computerised, telephone, or biblio-therapeutic platforms. A key objective of the work of all brief forms of CBT focuses on 'skilling up' the person engaging in the therapy with the tools to control their feelings and challenge negative thoughts (Layard et al., 2007, p. 3).

RESEARCH AND EVIDENCE SUPPORTING BCBT

BCBT is commonly utilised in the treatment of anxiety and low mood/mild depression in adults in primary care services. BCBT is an approach that compresses much of the traditional CBT work into fewer sessions. Essentially, the evidence for or against a treatment modality relies on the outcome and one has to be realistic in the projected outcomes for a brief form of therapy, especially if the presentation is inherently complex and long term. BCBT is generally not recommended for use with people with more complicated difficulties (e.g. complex trauma histories). This is due to the complicated relational difficulties people with interpersonal trauma histories can experience and the integrative and transdiagnostic approach required for trauma-informed care. However, BCBT-type interventions may be of use with such clients as part of a therapeutic intervention with a specific, short-term goal. Bond and Dryden (2008) canvassed a range of researchers and found that BCBT was probably most effective with less severe problems, and could produce both short- and long-term positive outcomes.

Recent evidence has argued that BCBT has a positive outcome in a varied range of presentations: in treating anxiety and depression (Cape et al., 2010; McHugh et al., 2013), binge eating (Fischer et al., 2014) and depression due to homesickness in international students (Saravanan et al., 2017). Importantly, BCBT has been used successfully with anxiety and depression where comorbid presentations exist, including veterans with physical health problems and anxiety and depression (Cully et al., 2017), cancer-related PTSD with comorbid anxiety/depression (Kangas et al., 2014) and insomnia with people experiencing depression, some of whom described suicidal thoughts (Pigeon et al., 2017).

Such a range of positive uses in practice suggests that researchers are continually pushing the use of shorter-term therapies to treat more complicated problems (if not in total, in part), and are generating data that will guide future practice. Such work is now challenging the historic notion that BCBT is only of use in less complicated presentations, but much more evidence is needed.

DELIVERING BCBT IN PRACTICE

Throughout this chapter, the use of BCBT is illustrated by use of case studies and repeated reference to the structure and organisation of practice and interventions.

STRUCTURE OF BCBT

An important factor in BCBT is that not all therapists may be both confident and sufficiently skilled in applying such a structured treatment. The therapist needs skills in motivating the client to address tasks and engage in exercises, and yet be sufficiently knowledgeable to maintain the therapeutic alliance. Often in CBT, attempts to identify automatic thoughts that are associated with problems are difficult to elicit. A refocusing on the emergent emotions and an exploration of personal meaning for the emotion can help unearth any automatic thoughts.

STRUCTURE OF THERAPY FOR EACH SESSION (TEMPLATE EXEMPLAR)

Table 1.1 Template exemplar for each session of BCBT

Start session and check client's problem(s)

Brief review of the past week

Agenda setting for the present session

Link work and feedback to previous session

Homework review

Discussion of agenda items

Homework setting

Check understanding and gain feedback for the session

The template from practice in Table 1.1 has clear links with Young and Beck's (1980) Cognitive Therapy Manual. The application of the structure is embedded into the process of therapy for each session.

PROCESS OF THERAPY (EXEMPLAR)

Table 1.2 Exemplar for the process of BCBT over eight sessions

Session	Content	Potential work
1	Introduce to CBT model Assess client and their concerns regarding treatment Set initial treatment plan	Developing a therapeutic relationship with orientation to the BCBT model. Establish an agenda (used in each session). Start to develop a collaborative formulation-type approach related to problems. Establish initial goals for therapy. Explore what the client understands about the problem they have and consider treatment options (potentially some psychoeducation work and eliciting a thought record). Homework (set in each session).
2	Continue to assess client and address concerns Establish collaborative goals for treatment Begin treatment	Ensure some level of engagement in the model and therapy. Continue with formulation and goal setting. Explore further understanding of treatment approaches and knowledge regarding problem (revisit the psychoeducation work and eliciting a thought record). Move on to more focused work on specific thoughts and beliefs – monitoring of these thoughts is part of the therapy. Explore the use of relaxation and behavioural activation-type work.
3	Continue treatment	Explore thoughts and assumptions in more detail and potential eliciting of core beliefs. Look at thoughts (maladaptive and automatic).
4	Continue treatment and review goals	Explore progress made and revisit assumptions and core beliefs. Look at any cognitive distortions. Utilise Socratic-type questions and thought records. Look at evidential-type work related to problems and the continuation of such.
5	Continue treatment	Reviewing progress will establish the timing of shifts in treatment.

Session	Content	Potential work
6	Continue treatment	Look at management of thoughts and consequences on behaviours. Revisit changes in thinking and the outcome on problems identified.
7	Continue treatment and explore ending of work and focus on how to maintain the changes made	Review changes made and start to focus on ending therapy. For example, look at a way to maintain the changes made. Explore learning. Start to identify and construct a relapse prevention package (inventory).
8	End treatment and refocus on maintaining improvement	Revisit previous work and firm up the relapse prevention package (inventory). Signpost to other agencies and/or resources. Make sure to address concerns and listen to worries from the client.

Although the process and skills are very similar to traditional CBT, with the briefer format there is more of an emphasis on key components: goal and agenda setting, collaboration, assessment, formulation and homework.

GOAL SETTING

At the outset, suitable goals that can be met in the short timeframe available need to be established. Consequently, SMART (specific, measureable, achievable, realistic and time-limited) goals are encouraged, and interventions are directed towards the achievement of these goals.

AGENDA SETTING

An agenda facilitates the efficient use of limited sessions by offering a structure that emphasises activity and progress to an agreed point. Agenda setting also demonstrates to clients that they have been heard and given an opportunity to talk about issues that are important to them.

COLLABORATION

Collaboration is a process of the client and therapist working together to address the goals of the therapeutic work. In many forms of therapy, the collaborative relationship can be neglected and to some it is seen as a technique instead of an inherent skill. Without collaboration, the therapy can become too directive and one-directional.

ASSESSMENT AND FORMULATION

Introduced from the first session, assessment and formulation aim to identify and map key problems and maintenance factors in order to inform subsequent treatment planning and goal-directed interventions. However, the formulation (mapping) is only as good as the information that drives it, so an accurate assessment of the problems is a key element for positive therapeutic outcomes. Therapists need to identify quickly the best route to establish what is happening and the assessment can follow various avenues and include information from standardised assessment tools. Some simplistic formulations adopt an ABC (Antecedent, Behaviour and Consequence) approach. Such an approach enables the client to quickly understand the way things are interlinked, but that behaviours can be shaped by both the antecedent and consequential thoughts or feelings.

A crucial difference in formulations in BCBT, as compared to CBT, is in the need to establish an accurate formulation quickly. However, both can use a simple snapshot of aspects related to an event (an example is shown in Figure 1.1) to enable the client to become comfortable with the model.

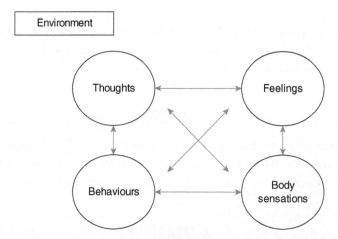

Figure 1.1 A workable example of a 'Hot Cross Bun' for both BCBT and CBT practice

Source: Greenberger and Padesky (1995)

HOMEWORK

Homework aims to consolidate the work engaged in and the goals for the session. Much of the content of homework relies upon the experience of the therapist and their knowledge of the process of treatment and the evidence base that exists for the problem under scrutiny. Commonly, the homework will involve tasks related to the last session (e.g. behavioural experiments), where the client will engage in some activity that will test out a frame of belief in a live setting. Homework can also be something as straightforward as recording thoughts or even psychoeducation, where a client may read something about their problems or the practicalities of BCBT.

SKILLS NEEDED TO CONDUCT BCBT

The therapeutic style utilised in BCBT is very different from counselling or analytical approaches. The relationship is highly collaborative and is considered a key component of the therapy rather than the main vehicle for change. Within BCBT, there is a focus on working together on jointly agreed problems and goals. The partnership is considered an equal one, where the therapist brings expertise of a range of theories, skills and knowledge while the client brings the expertise of their own lived experiences, skills and resources.

INTERVENTIONS

The interventions used in BCBT are very similar to traditional CBT, although they have a much tighter timeframe for completion and rely heavily on the client's active participation. Importantly, a clear explanation of the number of sessions and the formulation/goal-driven approach is a characteristic. Interventions, for example, include cognitive restructuring, behavioural activation, relaxation, problem solving and psychoeducation.

CLIENT ROLE

One of the challenges of BCBT is in the profile of who may benefit from it. Although utilising a similar approach to traditional CBT-type work (engaging in treatment both during and after sessions), clients engaging in the briefer format need to accept more responsibility, be more focused and motivated to change, and have an expectation that they will adopt an active learning style towards material both inside and outside sessions.

THERAPIST ROLE

The therapist probably needs to play a more active and directive role in BCBT, as compared to CBT, within sessions, while maintaining a style which encourages the collaboration that will be required to maximise the benefits of a short-term approach. Within BCBT, there is a greater need for the therapist to take responsibility for keeping sessions focused and goal-directed. The therapist needs to feel comfortable when directing clients back to the therapeutic tasks while simultaneously maintaining a strong working alliance. This can prove difficult for novice therapists who often lack the confidence and skills needed to do this or for therapists who have been previously oriented in person-centred approaches.

——————————— STORIES FROM PRACTICE ———————————

General practitioner (GP) referral

Peter is a 49-year-old man who has worked in a bank for 20 years and has experienced anxiety and depressive problems throughout his adult life. He was referred for therapy by his GP and was told it would be a brief series of sessions to help him address personal

(Continued)

difficulties experienced both before and after taking sickness leave from work. He wondered how this might help him as he had tried a longer version of therapy in the past and that had not helped.

Peter's scepticism about the shortened format of therapy was addressed by the therapist, who explained the BCBT model and invited him to collaborate and be active in his treatment. Working together towards Peter's goals for treatment helped to establish an effective thera-peutic alliance. Using skills that can be seen in the *Cognitive Therapy Scale Rating Manual* (Young & Beck 1980), the therapist carefully used the more generic skills (collaboration, feedback, understanding), which are more closely aligned with Rogerian skills (genuineness, active listening and empathy), but also the more specific skills aimed at arriving at an ini-tial formulation for the presenting problem. Importantly, the therapist utilised an agenda to organise the session and to provide a framework to enable adherence to the goals that Peter wanted to address in a smooth and orderly way.

The therapist made notes about the discussion to help set the agenda and, using the original Williams and Garland (2002) 5-areas assessment, helped to recognise and clarify the interlink-ing presentation of his problems (see Figure 1.2). Peter and the therapist agreed on eight 50-minute sessions. The aim was to enable Peter to start to talk about his problem(s) and then to start to make the links between his thinking at the time, his emotions, physical state and behaviour. Identifying alterations in these enabled the first debate related to a formulation.

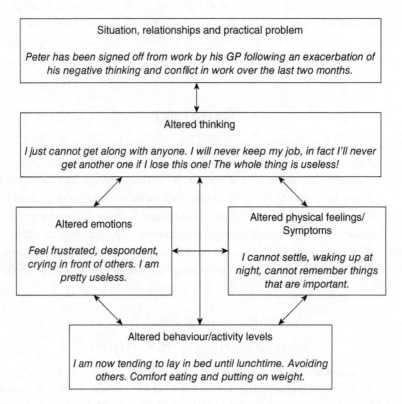

Figure 1.2   5-areas assessment for Peter at the first meeting

Source: Williams & Garland, 2002

Occupational setting referral

Martin is a 27-year-old man who is finding it very difficult to control his temper both inside and outside work. He has received a number of warnings from his manager. He was informed during his most recent performance review that any further incidents would result in discipli-nary action. He was directed to his company employee assistance programme (EAP), where he was offered a choice of counselling or CBT. Martin had previously experienced counselling and wanted to try a more structured approach.

The EAP authorised six 50-minute treatment sessions. Martin presented with a number of interrelated issues: frustration, leading to a loss of temper (shouting at his wife and destruc-tive behaviour), anxiety related to his job, and a perceived inability to adapt to new working systems. This had left him feeling low and overwhelmed.

The therapist considered Martin suitable for BCBT, given his motivation to engage, his ability to access his thoughts and feelings, and his willingness to engage in tasks outside the sessions. Treatment began with an assessment using some formal measures: the Patient Health Questionnaire (PHQ-9, Kroenke et al., 2001), the Generalised Anxiety Disorder Assessment (GAD-7, Spitzer et al., 2006), a semi-structured interview using Socratic questioning, and a functional analysis.

Martin and the therapist discussed treatment priorities and established SMART treatment goals to help them use the limited sessions effectively. They decided to focus on his frustra-tion and anger issues as these were influencing his relationships, and thus contributing to his anxiety and low mood.

Martin and his therapist used problem maintenance cycles to formulate the problem(s) and explore the relationship between his thoughts, feelings, behaviours and physical symptoms (Figure 1.3).

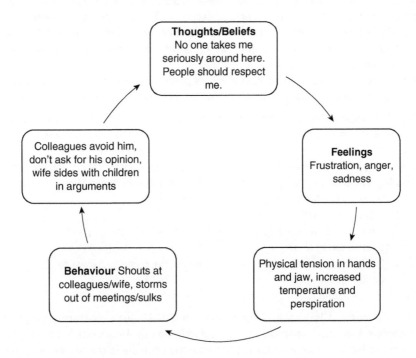

Figure 1.3 Maintenance cycle developed by Martin and the therapist

Interventions utilised within treatment were psychoeducation, relating to the role of perceptions and beliefs in the activation of anger, and relaxation training to help develop a level of awareness and management of Martin's arousal levels. Self-monitoring was used to aid the recognition of antecedents and consequences of anger, with cognitive restructuring to help generate alternative beliefs and an understanding of others' behaviour. In addition, skills training, including problem solving and assertiveness training, was used to help improve adaptive coping and communication. Martin considered the communication and assertiveness training to have the greatest impact on his progress.

Treatment concluded with relapse prevention and signposting to services and self-help material that would help Martin to work towards goals that were outside the parameters of the brief therapy programme.

Primary care setting referral

Anna is a 25-year-old woman who has found it difficult to get over a break-up with her partner eight months ago. She has been feeling increasingly low and depressed and has become withdrawn from friends, family and her usual activities. Anna contacted her GP after friends became worried about her. This was her first depressive episode of a mild to moderate nature. NICE Guidelines (2009) recommend a brief programme of CBT treatment. In Anna's case, this was provided by a primary care team within Anna's local medical practice.

NICE (2009) advocate the provision of individual, guided self-help based on CBT principles. Treatment includes written materials to support recovery as well as six face-to-face sessions over 9–12 weeks with a practitioner trained in delivering low-intensity CBT. The GP also prescribed a course of anti-depressant medication. Assessment included screening for risk (Cooper-Patrick et al., 1994) and standardised psychometric questionnaires (GAD-7, Spitzer et al., 2006; PHQ-9, Kroenke et al., 2001) as well as an exploration of predisposing and precipitating factors.

Anna and the therapist work on establishing a problem list and a set of therapeutic goals. Below is an example of a dialogue to demonstrate collaborative goal-setting with Anna:

THERAPIST: It will help if we can both share the same vision from our work together and what your goals and priorities are. What do you think you would like to gain from the work?

ANNA: Well, I'd like to feel happier and better about myself and my life.

THERAPIST: Great! That's a fantastic start. [Note that the therapist is taking any opportunity to provide positive encouragement from the outset.] If you were feeling better about yourself and your life what would you be doing differently?

ANNA: I would be more active and get out more.

THERAPIST: What sort of things would you do? [The therapist is using open Socratic questions to elicit information.]

ANNA: Well, I would start going out with my friends again, going into town and maybe watching football again.

THERAPIST: Those sound like positive goals. How often would you go out?

Here the therapist is guiding Anna to develop SMART goals that are appropriate for the parameters of BCBT, enabling the conceptualisation of Anna's difficulties (Figure 1.4). Interventions included psychoeducation to help Anna understand the nature of depression, its development and maintenance, behavioural activation, including activity scheduling to encourage engagement in adaptive and positively reinforcing activities, thought diaries and cognitive restructuring to address negative beliefs.

Treatment ended with an evaluation of outcomes and relapse prevention.

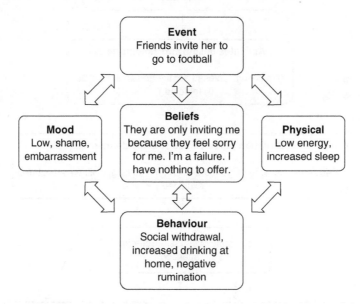

Figure 1.4 5-area formulation (note the slight change from the Williams & Garland (2002) 5-areas assessment) as applied to Anna's presentation

Source: Williams & Chellingsworth, 2010

Private referral

Aisha is a 19-year-old woman who has always thought of herself as an anxious person who is shy and lacks social skills. Bullying during her primary school years has left her feeling socially inadequate. She has developed an avoidant strategy (safety behaviour) for managing her anxiety. Recently, her anxiety has become harder to manage. Her manager has indicated she will soon be involved in a project that will necessitate socialising inside and outside work, the prospect of which fills her with dread. She is continually imagining worst-case scenarios relating to the forthcoming work and her physiological symptoms are increasingly uncontrollable.

Rather than speaking with her GP, Aisha contacted a private therapist who has been recommended by a family member. After an initial telephone consultation with the therapist, an agreement for 6–8 sessions of weekly CBT was contracted. The therapist assessed Aisha for her suitability for CBT (Safran et al., 1993), any risk factors, problem development and maintenance, social support and personal resources. Assessment tools included the CORE-10 (Barkham et al., 2013), GAD-7 (Spitzer et al., 2006) and the Liebowitz Social Anxiety Scale (LSAS, Liebowitz, 1987). All were utilised in conjunction with information from the interview and the *DSM-V* (American Psychiatric Association, 2013) criteria indicated moderate symptoms of social anxiety. Aisha was motivated and had good insight into her problems. With the therapist, she formulated these using the model adapted from Clark and Wells (1995) (see Figure 1.5).

(Continued)

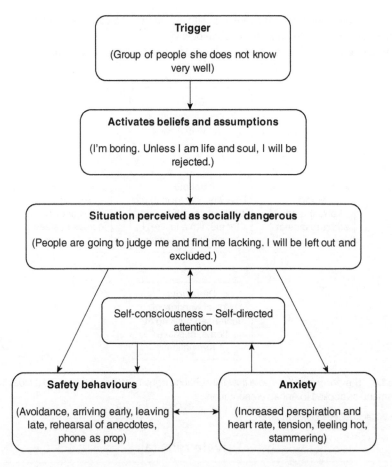

Figure 1.5 Adaptation of Clark and Wells (1995), as applied to Aisha's presentation

They compressed key interventions into the limited sessions and focused on social situations that would help Aisha achieve her short-term goals. Interventions included socialisation to the cognitive behavioural model, modification of safety behaviours to enable a disconfirmation of beliefs, shifting the focus of attention to enable an accurate processing of external events, video feedback to correct distorted negative self-images, verbal reattribution, and behavioural experiments to test beliefs and assumptions. A blueprint was developed which included an examination of how setbacks (the re-emergence of a noticeable increase in anxiety and safety behaviours) could be addressed (using a relapse prevention plan) in the future should they arise.

When Aisha had to engage with people in social situations she commonly avoided making conversation by looking away and focusing on her mobile phone, as though in conversation. She viewed the resultant lack of contact as a consequence of her actions. The aim of the action was to look busy and reduce the opportunity for people to speak to her and potentially negatively judge her. The lack of contact was seen as a positive outcome and is often seen by people with social-type anxiety as a result of implementing a safety behaviour. Aisha commented that 'by looking busy on my phone I avoided people making conversations and therefore getting to know me and then negatively judging me'. The use of the behaviour enabled Aisha to avoid the anxiety-provoking event.

The modification to Aisha's behaviour was to teach her simple, stress-reducing techniques, such as breathing exercises, and to select one of her safety behaviours, potentially the use of her mobile phone, to work on. Part way through the social event Aisha was to put the phone in her pocket and evaluate any social contact made. She would have the skills to reduce her stress by using the breathing exercises and would be asked to focus on the content of any conversation engaged in and, later, to evaluate the exact nature of the conversation. The aim was not to remove the mobile phone but to control its use as an aide to avoid contact with others, and to report on the actual content of conversation instead of her perception of its content.

Referral for claustrophobia via a charity

Patrick was a 45-year-old man who had struggled with claustrophobia for years. He had great difficulty in confined spaces (for example, in lifts, small, windowless rooms and buses). Patrick found his prospects were challenged; he had forgone promotion at work due to having to travel on the London underground system. At times, he found the problem tiresome and exhausting, having to adapt his life to avoid feared situations.

Patrick's search for psychological help was triggered by a forthcoming appointment for a Magnetic Resonance Imaging (MRI) scan. His physician considered the scan was essential to assess the state of his physical health and determine the best course of treatment. Patrick acknowledged the appointment was important and had contacted a local charity for help with his claustrophobic problem.

The scan was due in one month and the therapist emphasised the extent to which Patrick would need to be self-motivated outside the sessions in order to meet his goals. The therapist decided to use treatment based on Craske, Anthony and Barlow (2006), incorporating aspects of Öst's (2012) one-session phobia treatment. Patrick and the therapist scheduled four meetings prior to the MRI appointment, and agreed that some of their sessions may extend beyond the traditional therapeutic hour.

Treatment involved an initial assessment interview which used the standardised organisational measures, the Patient Health Questionnaire (PHQ-9, Kroenke et al., 2001) and the Generalised Anxiety Disorder Assessment (GAD-7, Spitzer et al., 2006). In addition, it used the Claustrophobia Questionnaire (CLQ, Radomsky et al., 2001) to gain further problem-specific information, and the *DSM-V* (American Psychiatric Association, 2013) to guide diagnosis. The use of a standardised tool such as the PHQ-9 or GAD-7 presented various opportunities to enhance practice. For the therapist, the tools created a baseline from which a change in symptoms could be evaluated, but also allowed the therapist to evaluate the narrative content of the session against the standardised assessment tool. Commonly, the use of the tools allows similar questions to be asked in slightly different ways. For the client, the tools also offer a baseline to which they can self-monitor improvement, but they also highlight areas for intervention that can be factored in to any plan of care. Such information can demystify the rationale for specific elements and goals engaged in within the therapeutic session.

The therapist collated detailed information relating to Patrick's beliefs and the identification of his maintenance factors. The therapist also provided information about the rationale

(Continued)

and content of the treatment, taking the opportunity to explore Patrick's worries about his MRI scan and the treatment. The therapist reassured Patrick that although the treatment would involve facing his fears and an initial increase in discomfort, the work would be controlled within his zone of tolerance.

Patrick stated that he only wanted to be able 'to handle' the scan at this moment, but accepted that, given that the scan constituted one of his greatest fears, it was likely that lesser fears might also be addressed even though these were not being targeted directly.

Patrick's treatment included the construction of a fear hierarchy to include the most anxiety-arousing situations and use of a series of exposure experiments to target the belief (e.g. entering a small room and locking the door). Patrick helped in the planning in order to enhance his sense of control and was encouraged to rate his subjective units of distress (SUDs) throughout the exposure. This helped the therapist to monitor the session and prevent Patrick from engaging in subtle cognitive avoidance during the task. The homework focused on Patrick educating himself about the air capacity that different rooms hold, the properties of airflow, and undertaking daily exposure tasks in line with his hierarchy. Cognitive restructuring examined the likelihood of suffocating in enclosed spaces and the evidence for and against this belief. Patrick made sufficient progress to be able to tolerate the idea of the scan.

TOP TIPS

- Establish the suitability of the client (and their needs) for BCBT.
- Work collaboratively towards realistic agreed goals in the time available.
- Use formulation to help inform efficient treatment planning.

EVALUATION OF THE STRENGTHS AND LIMITATIONS OF BCBT

The ability to deliver briefer formats of CBT has advantages, including cost-effectiveness and quick goal-directed and effective treatment. However, the access to psychological interventions remains inadequate with one in ten people in the UK waiting over a year to receive treatment and over half waiting three months to receive treatment (Mind, 2013). Accessibility to mental health services is a critical issue given the extent of harm that results from long waiting times. Consequences can be detrimental to familial, social and occupational functioning, and devastating to individuals, their communities and society as a whole.

Demand for mental health services is outpacing the availability of resources in many health service and third-sector organisations. Research has highlighted that BCBT can be delivered in a variety of formats and by a range of health professionals, offering the potential to disseminate and democratise much-needed access to a popular, evidence-based approach.

The shorter recovery times afforded by BCBT can provide reductions in distress levels and a quicker return to wellbeing and functioning, with the associated benefits this offers.

Where clients experience rapid treatment gains, the motivation to engage in further treatment is enhanced and the credibility of treatment is improved (Hazlett-Stevens & Craske, 2002).

In settings where clients are already burdened with ongoing medical appointments (e.g. for long-term health conditions), which in themselves act as stressors, reducing clinical visits offers further advantages, especially if briefer formats of CBT can be incorporated through the services already accessed.

FUTURE DIRECTIONS

There is a need to balance the appeal of BCBT with further research exploring the maintenance of acceptable outcomes. There are clear gaps in research related to the optimal number of sessions, session length, intensity, therapist training and issues such as model fidelity and use of manuals, self-help materials and other resources.

CBT's (and BCBT's) commitment to empirical testing means that research, especially component analyses and dismantling studies, will no doubt continue to focus on refining our current understanding of how specific mechanisms of change impact on recovery. Such a focus will inform the development of treatments that are likely to produce outcomes that are more efficacious.

PRACTITIONER TAKE HOME MESSAGES

- BCBT can offer therapeutic input where resources are limited.
- BCBT can potentially democratise the accessibility of evidence-based treatments.
- Some brief treatments appear to offer similar benefits to longer-term treatments.
- BCBT can be delivered in a variety of formats by a range of health professionals.

CONCLUSION

Adapting traditional delivery methods to incorporate briefer formats demonstrates that CBT is an incredibly versatile treatment. Brevity has clear advantages where resources are limited both for service providers and for clients. The demand for improving access to efficacious treatment is driving the increasingly innovative development, application and testing of new, briefer treatment protocols. Demand for BCBT approaches is showing no signs of slowing down and it is imperative, therefore, that the appetite for research to underpin this development is commensurate with the task.

Research is just beginning to explore the use of shorter therapies to treat increasingly more complex problems, thus far with mixed results. Findings from studies using BCBT to address comorbid presentations is challenging the previously held notions of the applicability of the approach. While many studies look to compare BCBT with waiting-list conditions, there is a need for further, well-designed trials to compare BCBT with standard CBT, especially for the more complex and arguably more real-world representative conditions where research is currently lacking.

─── DISCUSSION QUESTIONS ───

1. In what ways is BCBT different from traditional CBT?
2. What settings hold most evidence for the best use of BCBT?
3. What skills would someone using BCBT need to develop?
4. What structural and process factors are inherent in effective BCBT?

─── KEY TERMS ───

Behavioural activation A set of actions that aim to increase client activity while reinforcing factors that are improving the client's mood and functioning.

Bibliotherapy The use of reading material in the treatment of mental health and emotional-type problems, which is directed for a therapeutic purpose.

Cognitive restructuring The identification of problematic thoughts (e.g. all-or-nothing thinking) and subsequent modification of these as the client learns to understand the role of thinking in the maintenance of mood states.

Relaxation techniques Aim to reduce the physical arousal related to stress or worry. There are many different relaxation techniques, but most are easy to learn and are highly effective. The most common forms include muscular relaxation (where successive muscles are tightened and relaxed in a prescribed pattern) and breathing techniques which work to reduce physiological symptoms of anxiety.

Thought diary An important information-gathering tool that is used in establishing the role of thinking in the client's presenting problems but also as a monitoring tool to check progress.

─── FURTHER READING ───

Curwen, B., Palmer, S. & Ruddell, P. (2018) *Brief Cognitive Behaviour Therapy* (2nd ed.). London: Sage.

REFERENCES

American Psychiatric Association (2013) *Diagnostic and Statistical Manual of Mental Disorders* (5th ed.). Arlington, VA: American Psychiatric Publishing.

Barkham, M., Bewick, B., Mullin, T., Gilbody, S., Connell, J., Cahill, J., Mellor-Clark, J., Richards, D., Unsworth, G. & Evans, C. (2013) The CORE-10: A short measure of psychological distress for routine use in the psychological therapies. *Counselling and Psychotherapy Research, 13*(1), 3–13.

Bond, F.W. & Dryden, W. (2008) *Handbook of Brief Cognitive Behaviour Therapy*. Chichester: Wiley.

Cape, J., Whittington, C., Buszewicz, M., Wallace, P. & Underwood, L. (2010) Brief psychological therapies for anxiety and depression in primary care: Meta-analysis and meta-regression. *BMC Medicine, 8*, 38.

Clark, D.M. & Wells, A. (1995) A cognitive model of social phobia. In R. Heimberg, M. Liebowitz, D.A. Hope & F.R. Schneier (Eds.), *Social Phobia: Diagnosis, Assessment and Treatment* (pp. 69–93). New York: Guilford Press.

Cooper-Patrick, L., Crum, R.M. & Ford, D.E. (1994) Identifying suicidal ideation in general medical patients. *JAMA, 272*(22), 1757.

Craske, M. G., Antony, M. M. & Barlow, D. H. (2006) *Mastering Your Fears and Phobias* (2nd ed.). New York: Oxford University Press.

Cully, J.A., Stanley, M.A., Petersen, N.J., Hundt, N.E., Kauth, M.R., Naik, A.D., Sorocco, K., Sansgiry, S., Zeno, D. & Kunik, M.E. (2017) Delivery of brief cognitive behavioral therapy for medically ill patients in primary care: A pragmatic randonised clinical trial. *Journal of Internal Medicine, 32*(9), 1014–1024.

Curwen, B., Palmer, S. & Ruddell, P. (2018) *Brief Cognitive Behaviour Therapy* (2nd ed.). London: Sage.

Fischer, S., Meyer, A.H., Dremmel, D., Schlup, B. & Munsch, S. (2014) Short-term cognitive behavioral therapy for binge eating disorder: Long-term efficacy and predictors of long-term treatment success. *Behavior Research and Therapy, 58*, 36.

Greenberger, D. & Padesky, C. (1995) *Mind Over Mood: A Cognitive Therapy Treatment Manual for Clients*. New York: Guilford Press.

Hazlett-Stevens, H. & Craske, M.G. (2002) Brief cognitive-behavioral therapy: Definition and scientific foundations. In F. Bond & W. Dryden (Eds.), *Handbook of Brief Cognitive Behaviour Therapy*. Chichester: Wiley.

Kangas, M., Milross, C. & Bryant, R.A. (2014) A brief, early cognitive-behavioral program for cancer-related PTSD, anxiety, and comorbid depression. *Cognitive Behavioral Practice, 21*, 416–431.

Kroenke, K., Spitzer, R.L. & Williams, J.B.W. (2001) The PHQ-9: Validity of a brief depression severity measure. *Journal of General Internal Medicine, 16*(9), 606–613.

Layard, R., Clark, D., Bell, S., Knapp, M., Meacher, B., Priebe, S., Turnberg, L., Thornicroft, G. & Wright, B. (2006) The depression report: A new deal for depression and anxiety disorders. *The Centre for Economic Performance's Mental Health Policy Group*. London: LSE.

Layard, R., Clark, D., Knapp, M. & Mayraz, G. (2007) Cost–benefit analysis of psychological therapy. *National Institute Economic Review, 202*, 90–98.

Liebowitz, M.R. (1987) Social phobia. *Modern Problems in Pharmacopsychiatry, 22*, 141–173.

McHugh, P., Brennan, J., Galligan, N., McGonagle, C. & Byrne, M. (2013) Evaluation of a primary care adult mental health service: Year 2. *Mental Health in Family Medicine, 10*(1), 53–59.

Mind (2013) We still need to talk: A report on access to talking therapies. www.mind.org.uk/media/494424/we-still-need-to-talk_report.pdf.

NICE. (2009) Depression in adults: Recognition and management. *Clinical guideline* [CG90]. https://www.nice.org.uk/guidance/cg90.

Öst, L.G. (2012) One-session treatment: Principles and procedures with adults. In T.E. Davis (III), T.H. Ollendick & L.G. Öst (Eds.), *Intensive One-Session Treatment of Specific Phobias* (pp. 59–96). New York: Springer.

Pigeon, W.R., Funderburk, J., Bishop, T.M. & Crean, H.F. (2017) Brief cognitive behavioral therapy for insomnia delivered to depressed veterans receiving primary care services: A pilot study. *Journal of Affective Disorders, 217*, 105–111.

Radomsky, A.S., Rachman, S., Thordarson, D.S., McIsaac, H.K. & Teachman, B.A. (2001) The claustrophobia questionnaire. *Journal of Anxiety Disorders, 15*, 287–297.

Safran, J.D., Segal, Z.V., Vallis, T.M., Shaw, B.F. & Samstag, L.W. (1993) Assessing patient suitability for short-term cognitive therapy with an interpersonal focus. *Cognitive Therapy and Research, 17*(1), 23–38.

Saravanan, C., Alias, A. & Mohamad, M. (2017) The effects of brief individual cognitive behavioural therapy for depression and homesickness among international students in Malaysia. *Journal of Affective Disorders, 220*, 108–116.

Spitzer, R.L., Kroenke, K., Williams, J.B.W. & Löwe, B. (2006) Brief measure for assessing generalized anxiety disorder: The GAD-7. *Archives of Internal Medicine, 166*(10), 1092–1097.

Williams, C. & Chellingsworth, M. (2010) *CBT: A Clinician's Guide to Using the Five Areas Approach.* London: Hodder Arnold.

Williams, C. & Garland, A. (2002) A cognitive–behavioural therapy assessment model for use in everyday clinical practice. *Advances in Psychiatric Treatment, 8*(3), 172–179.

Young, J. & Beck, A.T. (1980) *Cognitive Therapy Scale Rating Manual*, www.beckinstitute.org.

2

TIME-LIMITED PERSON-CENTRED THERAPY

DIMITRIOS MONOCHRISTOU

INTRODUCTION

In this chapter, we will explore a brief approach to person-centred therapy (PCT), describing how PCT can be implemented in a time-limited therapeutic context. The main topics we will cover in this chapter are:

- What is person-centred therapy and where does it come from?
- What does time-limited person-centred therapy look like?
- How does brief PCT work in practice?

THEORETICAL INTRODUCTION OF PERSON-CENTRED THERAPY

Person-centred therapy is an approach to psychotherapy and counselling developed by Carl Rogers in the 1940s. As a theory, it is rooted in humanism, a movement proposing that subjective human experience is central in trying to understand people, and that human beings have a self-actualising tendency, rather than psychopathology. The term *self-actualisation* is used in humanism to describe the inherent nature of human beings to gravitate towards fulfilling their potential and leading fulfilling lives. Self-actualisation is the ultimate phase of development in Abraham Maslow's hierarchy of needs, which is possible when a person has their basic survival, emotional and social needs met (Maslow, 1943).

Other key theorists of the humanism movement have included Rollo May, Viktor Frankl and Irvin Yalom.

In addition to humanism, PCT embraces a phenomenological philosophy, which is a philosophical approach developed by the philosophers Edmund Husserl and Martin Heidegger. Phenomenology focuses on a person's interpreted meaning of their subjective (rather than the objective) experience. Overall, the key principle of PCT is that positive change in a person's emotional experience can occur in a therapeutic space when a safe and trusting relationship is developed between the client and the therapist. The nature of this relationship was defined by Rogers through six core conditions, which describe how to achieve constructive change in therapy:

1. Two persons are in psychological contact.
2. The first, whom we shall term the client, is in a state of incongruence, being vulnerable or anxious.
3. The second person, whom we shall term the therapist, is congruent or integrated in the relationship.
4. The therapist experiences unconditional positive regard for the client.
5. The therapist experiences an empathic understanding of the client's internal frame of reference and endeavors to communicate this experience to the client.
6. The communication to the client of the therapist's empathic understanding and unconditional positive regard is to a minimal degree achieved. (Rogers, 1957, pp. 95–96)

The idea of adopting these relational principles in therapy is to encourage the exploration of the client's experience of life in order to increase their awareness of their feelings, wishes, needs and values, in contrast to those imposed upon them through cultural and societal narratives. The ultimate outcome of the PCT process will be for the client to make life choices based on their own sense of meaning within the wider context of their social and cultural environment. In the end, their self-narrative will comprise their own values and those environmental elements integrated, welcomed and accepted within the client.

CHANGE AS HAPPENING IN A MOMENT IN TIME

Central to the PCT culture and philosophy is the premise that the therapeutic encounter cannot be medicalised and manualised; it must be built within the safety of the therapeutic relationship. Therefore, time-limited PCT is not suitable for everyone, particularly those who may need longer to feel safe developing therapeutic relationships (Feltham, 1995). However, time-limited PCT can work well in a number of situations, including when a client wishes to focus on a specific experience or phenomenon, or in *crisis* situations where a client has been faced with a sudden disruption of their current experience, even if this brings up issues from their past (Tudor, 2008).

There remains some debate as to the suitability of time-limited PCT among PCT theorists and practitioners, with some practitioners considering brief PCT to be contradictory to the essence of the approach, particularly when the time limit is externally imposed, thus obstructing the client's movement towards self-determination through personal choice. Some believe that counselling has succumbed to the demands of modern, fast-paced life to the detriment of the process of therapeutic and personal change (Thorne, 1999; Proctor et al., 2006). Often, current priorities in health and social care lead to a focus on tests of efficacy, value for money and a return on investments, which now make short-term therapies, including time-limited PCT, the only options of therapy for people to access. Consequently, although there can be many practical benefits to time-limited PCT, brief therapies can be seen as a response to an imperfect system, rather than a response to the needs of the clients.

Finally, the inevitability of externally imposed limits to therapy is not necessarily restricted to practical hurdles such as funding and the unavailability of resources. In existential therapies, which are related to humanistic approaches, becoming aware and living by certain limits in life is a step towards therapeutic progress and change (Van Deurzen, 2012; Cooper, 2015). For example, assuming the client can have absolute freedom to define their life is unrealistic and is perhaps an unhelpful expectation to be promoted through the therapeutic process. Similarly, the time limit in PCT can serve as a helpful platform for working within a boundaried timeframe, working towards a predictable ending, reinforcing the fact that limits are a natural part of life.

SETTING THE THERAPEUTIC SCENE

It is widely recognised that the therapeutic setting will influence the experience of therapy: for example, elements such as the waiting time for the appointment, the waiting area, the room decoration, how the client is welcomed into the room, the timing of the session, navigating punctuality, etc. Across time, PCT theorists Tudor (2008) and Taft (1933) have written about the therapeutic benefits of being conscious of time limits as a way of acknowledging and processing other limits in life as well. Working within a time limit and towards an ending can support the person to work through their resistance to address matters they cannot control and instead develop personal ways to cope with those realities. Therefore, learning that embraces the fact that life is not in its nature unrestricted can be made possible in the therapeutic encounter by being conscious of limitations.

Finally, it has also been considered in theory that positive change for the client can occur in the therapeutic contract regardless of the length of the therapeutic contract. Rogers himself (1959) discusses the nature and quality of a movement towards psychological change – a change in perception, an improved awareness of the client's situation – happening in a moment in time within the therapeutic relationship. O'Hara (1999) expands this by mentioning that psychological change can happen at any point in therapy, regardless of imposed time limits, as long as the aforementioned core conditions of PCT are in action. Similarly, Paul McGahey, a therapeutic practitioner (Tudor, 2008), explains that the quality of the therapeutic relationship between client and counsellor is central and that clients can make rapid changes when that relationship is in place.

THE EVIDENCE BASE AND EVALUATION

Aligning to the philosophy of PCT, that medicalising suffering and applying diagnostic labels can be unhelpful, we will explore the evidence base as a whole, rather than for specific diagnoses. Additionally, it is important to note that common mental health difficulties (e.g. anxiety and depression) are often the result of a multitude of experiences that lie beneath their label, for example, traumatic experiences and losses, shame, low self-esteem, and interpersonal skills, just to name a few.

Time-limited PCT can be helpful across a range of settings. In a qualitative study involving 50 case studies of PCT lasting three or four sessions, all clients self-reported having experienced empowerment, enhanced safety and insight (Timulak & Lietaer, 2001). In other words, participants reached significant goalposts in their journey of change, as conceptualised by PCT, so they could make choices and increase their awareness of their personal circumstances. Additionally, within a student counselling service, outcome measures showed consistent improvement, especially in the first four weeks of brief, non-directive, person-centred counselling (Cornelius-White, 2003). The clients in this study received a maximum of 16 sessions, although the average length of counselling was just under eight sessions, a finding that supports the effectiveness of time-limited person-centred counselling. This study shows that where clients could choose the length of their therapy, up to 16 sessions, they often decided that less than the maximum was enough. Further, time-limited PCT, between six and 12 sessions (average seven), has been found to lead to positive outcomes for clients with common mental health problems, such as anxiety and depression (Gibbard & Hanley, 2008). In this study, effectiveness was not limited to clients with mild to moderate distress, but also extended to people with long-term emotional difficulties.

Additionally, it is interesting to look at studies that have compared the effectiveness of PCT with other therapeutic modalities. Recently, outcomes between cognitive behavioural therapy (CBT) and time-limited PCT delivered to a sample of 33,243 clients experiencing depression across 103 Improving Access to Psychological Therapies (IAPT) services in the UK were compared (Pybis et al., 2017). CBT is a treatment recommended by the National Institute for Care Excellence (NICE) and used regularly in primary mental healthcare in the National Health Service (NHS). CBT emphasises working through thoughts and behaviours for the improvement of a person's emotional wellbeing. The study demonstrated that time-limited PCT generated clinically significant and reliable change when delivered to clients for between two and 10 sessions. The improvement rates were measured from self-assessment scores used in IAPT and primary care.

The effectiveness of PCT and CBT were comparable. The findings were welcomed by the British Association for Counselling and Psychotherapy (BACP) as influential for the improvement of the standing of brief PCT within statutory services and the therapeutic evidence base. Further, in a comparative study that delivered PCT to 1,709 clients from 32 NHS primary care services from 2002 to 2005 for an average of 6.82 sessions (Stiles et al., 2008), results showed that almost 76% of clients reported improvements in their emotional wellbeing. At the same time, the study found that PCT was equally effective compared to CBT and psychodynamic therapy. Psychodynamic therapy is a psychotherapeutic approach rooted in Freud's psychoanalysis and further developed by Carl Jung, Melanie Klein and other theorists of the field (see Chapter 8). Its focus is the uncovering of the unconscious to help the client work through psychological defences that have often been established in early life and form adaptive responses to their challenges.

A PRACTICAL GUIDE TO PCT

To understand how time-limited PCT operates, we need to look first at the nature of change that PCT claims to bring about for people, or the change that we as counsellors and therapists hope to see for clients that come to us for therapy. As discussed by Rogers (2003, 2004), there are some key outcomes we can observe within the PCT process. Table 2.1 presents my interpretation and structure around the movement of change as understood in PCT.

Table 2.1   Movement of change through time-limited PCT

Nature of change	Before	After
Named/un-named difficulties	Symptoms, externalising, past reference, objectification, fixed constructs	Self, introspection, feelings, relativity of constructs, present reference, personal values-evaluations
Perception of self	Fixed, negative, generalised, externally defined, emotional/ impulsive, influenced by past, divided, inadequate, undeserving	Changeable, positive, worthy, defined internally, reality based, influenced by present, integrated, resilient, accepting
Nature of perception	Abstractions, generalisations, absolute, unconditional, inflexible, unexamined, non-reflective, rigid	Specific, accurate, realistic, personal, relative, reflective, changeable
Awareness of denied experience	Habitual, externally defined, generalised, repression of evidence threatening established concepts, sedimentation of perceptions	Openness to experiences contradicting existing constructs, resilient to ensuing anxiety, discovering blind spots in perceptions, expansion to include new learning
Valuing process	Values introjected, external locus of evaluation, control, fixed, residing externally, habitual	Internal locus of evaluation, ownership, real self, loss/change of formerly held beliefs, alterable, residing in the self, new

Table 2.1 (Continued)

Nature of change	Before	After
Relationships	Need-centred, other-referential, high expressed emotion, non-reflective, ingenuine	Value-centred, mutual, genuine, honest, confident, appropriate emotive levels, self- and other- respectful
Behaviour	Sedimentation, repetition, internal tension, low distress tolerance, defensive, habitual	Break of dysfunctional behavioural cycles, willingness to alter dysfunctional patterns, tolerance

For these changes to take place in therapy, the therapist works through PCT processes to assist the client to uncover their genuine qualities and their authentic self. This can be a difficult process as our real wishes, needs and values can often be hidden beneath layers of our own awareness that have developed over the years in an effort to adapt to environmental factors, i.e. caregivers' personalities, teachers, friends, societal rules, etc. Hence, the counsellor will attempt to support the client to get in touch with feelings that have been unknown to them, elaborating, reflecting on and encouraging emotional expression and pointing out defensiveness against it. Becoming aware of and being able to see through the various 'façades' that are often used to obstruct their view of themselves will increase self-awareness and the integration of denied or ignored parts of the self within their personality. The challenge of this process lies with the fact that we are often unaware that these 'façades' exist within us. This tricks our minds into believing that the parts of the self that we have nurtured in order to be accepted by important people in our lives are in accordance with our genuine selves, which is not always the case.

Consequently, a person will become more open to their experiences and reality through the process of PCT and will develop faith in themselves, their values and qualities. This process facilitates self-evaluation and an awareness that people will always be in a state of process and movement, rather than fixed in time (Rogers, 2004).

TOP TIP

Don't cause yourself a headache trying to identify each of the above traits in every client you see. Personality and change express themselves differently in every person and context.

THE THERAPEUTIC RELATIONSHIP

In PCT, the main contributor to therapeutic change is considered to be the relationship that forms between client and therapist, characterised by the conditions of unconditional acceptance, empathy and congruence, and the authenticity of the therapist. Therefore, if a safe base is available, the client will gradually be able to *safely* explore their situation and openly discuss their awareness of their feelings and thoughts with the therapist, which may have been blocked previously. Within a safe and supportive relationship, the client will be able to accept themselves, try out behaviours and express feelings without feeling invalidated. Hence, the client will be empowered to model new possibilities for self-awareness and for relating to other people.

The therapist can facilitate this relational environment by responding to their clients' presence and verbalisations in certain ways. The therapist can do this by staying in their client's frame of reference by following their content and communicating this with the client without introducing their own views. Instead, the role of the therapist is to reflect back to their client the essence of the expressed meanings and feelings, not only cognitive content. This means that the client can be talking about something of the past, about another person, or about their thoughts and the skilled counsellor will point out to them their feelings, in the present moment, also known as the 'here and now' experience. For this process to be productive, which means well received by the client, the therapist will have to follow the client's pace, allowing appropriate silences and only responding when necessary. They will be communicating receptiveness, facilitating a safe environment for self-expression, and using warmth to show acceptance. The therapist will use clear and simple language, not scientific jargon, in order to ensure productive communication close to the client's experience. They will follow the client's lead without redirecting the discussion but trusting the client's internal process. They will also be natural, grounded and receptive to their own moment-to-moment experience and to their client's experience.

PRACTITIONER ATTUNEMENT

Being attuned to one's own experience is important for the counsellor. Self-aware and attuned practitioners can more readily understand their client's implicit communications and will not react with inappropriate emotion but will acknowledge any distressing feelings expressed by the client (Freire et al., 2013). The counsellor, just as any other human being, has their own subjective experiences of relating to other people and will have their own personal emotional responses to content brought by their client in the session. In order for the counsellor to be emotionally aligned with the client they will have to be able to contain their own personal reactions and be aware of their own material. That will help the counsellor to respond to their client with curiosity, appreciating the uniqueness of their experience and casting to one side assumptions regarding the situation of the client (Borg, 2013, p. 64).

TOP TIP —————

Working in this way can involve a lot of uncertainty as one is following the client into the unknown. Don't isolate yourself; be open about your practice with peers and your supervisor.

COLLABORATION AND AGREEING A FOCUS FOR THERAPY
DEVELOPING A THERAPEUTIC FOCUS

When it comes to time-limited PCT, Feltham and Dryden (2006) advocate the importance of agreeing a focus. This is also encapsulated in the principle of collaboration in the experiential literature, which encourages mutual involvement with the therapeutic tasks derived from a set focus (Sanders & Hill, 2014). For example, a client may be nipping in and out of their emotional exploration of certain events in their life because it is difficult for them to stay with it. The 'pure' person-centred counsellor would follow the client's process and point out that the client is doing exactly that. The person-centred counsellor who works within a time limit may do the former but also remind the client of their agreed focus and that staying with the emotional processing of the experience may achieve their therapeutic goals. There is no hard-and-fast rule as to the strength of the therapeutic relationship and many personal factors will define its nature.

INTEGRATING HUMANISTIC APPROACHES

Below I briefly describe some techniques that can be brought into PCT in certain therapeutic circumstances. The added skills are borrowed from experiential therapies such as Emotion-Focused Therapy, Focusing-Oriented Therapy and Solution-Oriented Therapy, which are also rooted in humanism and developed through the work of Leslie Greenberg, Eugene Gendlin and Steve de Shazer (Sanders, 2004; Tudor, 2008):

- *Difficulty – Stuckness*: The exploration of an experience may have reached a plateau in therapy. The counsellor may want to invite the client to turn to their embodied experience in the present, visualise it and work with that metaphor. For example, a client may visualise a difficult memory feeling like a big heavy boulder that they are carrying around and they wish they could for one moment put it down next to them and turn away or see it disintegrate, or become lighter and smaller, and so on.
- *Difficulty – The 'random' extra-therapeutic incident*: A client may be particularly upset about a particular event or situation outside therapy. The counsellor will invite the client to walk them through the event, step by step, as if it was happening in the present. Often, this leads to identifying emotional and behavioural patterns that connect to the client's original difficulties as people tend to have particular patterns of behaviour when faced with difficult situations.
- *Difficulty – Overwhelming feelings*: These may impede constructive exploration. The counsellor may attempt to ground the client by bringing them to the here and now. For example, the counsellor may invite the client to visualise a safe space or a visual anchor that has a soothing impact on the client. The client can be asked to put their difficult feelings in a box, or out of their view, etc.

- *Difficulty – A divided sense of self*: A client makes reference to parts of themselves – an old self, an ideal self, an angry or critical self, etc. The therapist may want to assist the client to get into dialogue with those parts of the self, to look at what they need, why they say what they say, what they are asking from the client, or to explore if there are any parts of the self that lie dormant (e.g. the forgiving self).
- *Difficulty – Discussing emotions*: The counsellor may invite the client to listen into their embodied experience to unblock feelings. There are some other techniques that may sit less comfortably with counsellors as they veer further away from the person-centred principle of non-directiveness. These are referred to in the literature as unlayering or unblocking. Repetitive questioning or instruction given on behalf of the therapist can be uncomfortable in a PCT context. For example, the therapist may ask the client to complete the following sentence sequence: *I feel… because… and this makes me feel….* This sequence is repeated until a shift transpires in the client's awareness or a realisation forms.

The experienced therapist will know when and how to introduce certain interventions so that they do not violate the client's ownership by directing the content or the process of therapy. Close supervision of the application of those techniques is crucial for them to become integrated into a counsellor's therapeutic model. The preservation of the depth of the relationship needs always be the primary consideration for the therapist.

TOP TIP

In the abundance of therapeutic activities that can be employed it can feel daunting to have to decide which is suitable. Always think about why you are making a certain intervention in counselling. In other words: 'Am I doing this for my client or for me?'

STORIES FROM PRACTICE

The following cases are adequately anonymised to protect the clients' identities. In time-limited PCT, the right balance will have to be achieved between client-led exploration and tentative suggestions by the counsellor in order to preserve the quality of the therapeutic relationship and not inhibit safe exploration and the potential for change. It is useful for the client and counsellor to have a conversation at the start of their contract about the number of sessions, what can be achieved, where to put the focus and how they will work. The client then feels active in the process. Furthermore, you will find in the case studies below the importance of timing and context in terms of when interventions are used. Again, timing ensures the client's frame of reference is always taken into account, which again promotes a trusting relationship between the two parties.

The first vignette has a beginning, middle and end to summarise the full therapeutic process; it is presented as a small session abstract to illustrate the use of specific suggestions by the counsellor to mobilise deeper processes.

David

David was a young man who came for counselling in order to express his anger and disappointment towards the health services, which he felt repeatedly let him down by not thoroughly investigating his chronic physical complaints. David was feeling acute pains in his upper back, abdomen and legs. He had been checked by his GP and specialist clinics and his doctors told him that the underlying reason for the pains must be psychological. David was not convinced and was frequently visiting the local hospital emergency department only to be sent back home. David said to me that the doctors were not bothered and considered him a 'pest'. He became increasingly frustrated and socially isolated as his confidence reduced due to feeling unimportant. He sought counselling with the local counselling service to address his emotional state and was referred to me.

We contracted to meet for seven weekly sessions. In a brief therapy model, I ask my clients what their expectations are from counselling. This is to identify if there is a specific area the client wants to concentrate on because a lack of focus can mean that the limited sessions can pass to little avail. In the words of David, he needed to 'offload' and he wished his quality of life would improve. He was feeling very tense, frustrated and consumed by his physical complaints. It made sense in the first two sessions to allow the space for David to get things off his chest. I used person-centred skills of active and empathic listening in order to help David feel safe and accepted in the counselling space. I reflected back thoughts and emotions so that he felt acknowledged and that his experience was one worth listening to. I summarised the verbal content he communicated to me, provided verbal and non-verbal encouragers and open-ended questions to prompt him to continue his introspection. Overall, I followed his train of thought with a warm demeanour and stayed with his frame of reference and pace. I wanted to allow him to feel in control, unlike how he had been feeling over the past few years.

After two sessions, David came to the third session in higher spirits. Frequent reviews of the counselling process are very important, especially in a time-limited setting. David said it felt good to get 'things out with somebody who listens' rather than to overthink alone. In brief counselling it can be useful to gently remind the client of the agenda they themselves set at the start. This led us to address his wellbeing. The client's own sense of direction will help with furnishing them with a tangible outcome and prevent an abrupt ending amid increased vulnerability. I told David that I was noticing that over the past few years he had been waiting to be helped by someone outside of him (i.e. the health services) whereas now, by coming to counselling, it seemed that he was taking matters into his own hands. He noticed that some things were out of his powers and even though he was wishing for a different treatment from his doctors, he acknowledged that he now needed to take more care of himself.

It felt appropriate to use some solution-focused questions in order to establish if David was in a place to think about what a future with an increased quality of life would look like. David was saying that he gets down when he is doing something that he normally enjoys but then a physical pain interferes and reminds him of his situation. I asked him what it would feel like if he was experiencing pain but had somehow managed to feel more relaxed about it. He acknowledged that it was the emotional aftermath of his pains that aggravated his situation and not the pains themselves. What was painful was to not be heard, which is something he had also experienced by his family and some friends. In sessions five and six, David reflected that he did not wish to be consumed by negative feelings about his perspective of his doctors being dismissive and he could now focus on the life he wanted to have. He managed to think of ways of being at peace with his pains through doing enjoyable things. We also explored ways in which he could resume some of his relationships.

In counselling, David managed to embark on a relationship with me where he wasn't dismissed. This happened through the application of relational skills that established conditions such as empathy and acceptance. David seemed to come out the other side more secure and motivated to improve his life; he managed to mobilise his internal direction (see Figure 2.1).

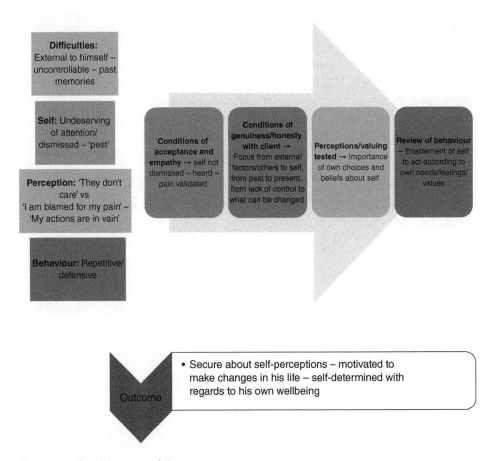

Figure 2.1   David's process of change

Grace

Grace sought counselling for her low mood and self-reported low self-esteem. In the first few sessions, she identified feelings of self-loathing and we explored the family dynamics that had been the basis 3for her self-perception. The following extract is from session 6:

GRACE (G):   One moment I think everything is going to be fine, I am keeping busy with the things I enjoy doing, the next minute I get so worried about the future, University, job prospects and I really feel I don't deserve any of it.

COUNSELLOR (C):   Part of you is optimistic while another part is very pessimistic.

My intention here was to point out the existence of two separate driving forces within her. This could potentially lead to us exploring both of them or getting them into dialogue when the time is right to diffuse the conflict between them.

G: Yes, and it's like I am constantly in and out of these different moods.

C: This sounds very unsettling.

My aim here was to validate her emotional experience.

G: It's disappointing really. Right when I think I am managing, this pessimism takes over and I am back where I started.

C: There seems to be a very real split in you between a hopeful 'you' that is managing well and another 'you' that slams the breaks. How would you feel about working on those opposing parts in yourself today?

Given this is session 6, I feel our relationship is strong enough for me to suggest an exercise. I still phrase it as to give her the opportunity to decline.

G: That makes sense.

C: What helps is to try and visualise the part that is causing you distress, the self-critical part in our case, and then attempt to engage in a dialogue with it. We will do this at your own pace and in the way that suits you best.

I am tentatively introducing the exercise and reassuring her that we will fit it around her needs. We then proceed with it:

G: OK, I am not sure how this will work but I came prepared to challenge myself anyway, so...

C: OK, let's start with thinking about your critical self. Can you think about what it looks like? Does it remind you of anyone – it can be a person, an animal or object or something from your imagination?

G: That's an easy one, it's definitely my parents, my mum has always tried to dissuade me from going to Uni. 'Get a real job out in the country just like we did'.

C: It seems like you have a really clear idea in your mind. How would you like us to refer to your critical self during this exercise?

G: Just 'mum', I think.

C: OK, so what is 'mum' saying to you when you feel down and pessimistic about your future?

G: 'I told you you weren't good enough to study, what are you trying to prove', it's like she's telling me I'm out here on my own and she's waiting for me to fail so I can be proven wrong and they are right, like 'give up already'...

C: OK, and what about your positive and content self? Can you describe it?

G: I can see it now, I am going about my business, reading my books, going for a run, being genuinely pleasant around my friends and not just faking it.

C: Great. So imagine now that you can talk to your negative self, to 'mum', what would you say in response?

G: 'Mum, we are so different, I know where you're coming from, but I'm not you. I know I'm going to make it, I have been doing alright so far, there's no reason I can't continue like that...'

The dialogue between the two 'selves' continued and helped Grace understand the more hopeful forces in herself and disarm her self-critical side as understandable due to her history, but unfounded based on her present experience.

CONCLUSION

Brief PCT prioritises the quality of the client–counsellor relationship and emphasises client self-determination. Through the application of certain therapeutic conditions, the client has the chance to develop an honest relationship with themselves, others and their world. The time limit offers the opportunity to focus on specific difficulties and for the practitioner to be creative in their approach by inserting appropriate experiential techniques into their practice. This can ensure that possibilities for exploration, expanding of awareness and change are not missed in a time-limited course of counselling.

DISCUSSION QUESTIONS

1. How can a non-directive model such as person-centred therapy justify the use of techniques that can be seen as directive, such as the ones described in this chapter?
2. How can the counsellor help the client to keep to the session focus without violating their self-determination?
3. What implications does the time limit have for the relationship between the client, the counsellor and a counselling service?

FURTHER READING

For more on the application of skills mentioned in this chapter I recommend:

- Sanders, P. & Hill, A. (2014) *Counselling for Depression: A Person-Centred and Experiential Approach to Practice*. London: Sage. This book presents the 'Counselling for Depression' model for time-limited counselling currently rolled out in the NHS IAPT services. The reader will find a structured and detailed working framework for the application of a time-limited (max. 20 sessions) person-centred and experiential model with case examples.
- Tudor, K. (2008) *Brief Person-centred Therapies*. London: Sage. This book describes how brief person-centred therapies can work with different client difficulties. It draws together person-centred and experiential therapies. It will help the reader to understand how brief person-centred therapy can be applied to a variety of client presentations.

For a detailed account of person-centred therapy and how it applies to practice:

- Mearns, D. & Thorne, B. (2013) *Person-Centred Counselling in Action*. London: Sage.

With regards to accepting the time limit in therapy as a way for the client to adjust to the idea of further limitations in life, such as the finiteness of life and lack of control over future events, the book below on existential counselling describes ways to integrate those concepts in therapeutic work:

- Van Deurzen, E. (2012) *Existential Counselling & Psychotherapy in Practice*. London: Sage.

The recommended interventions for mental health difficulties can be found on the website of the National Institute for Health and Care Excellence: www.nice.org.uk/guidance

REFERENCES

Borg, L.K. (2013) Holding, attaching and relating: A theoretical perspective on good enough therapy through analysis of Winnicott's good enough mother, using Bowlby's attachment theory and relational theory. *Theses, Dissertations, and Projects*, 588. Available at: https://scholarworks.smith.edu/theses/588

Cooper, M. (2015) *Existential Psychotherapy and Counselling: Contributions to a Pluralistic Practice*. London: Sage.

Cornelius-White, J.H.D. (2003) The effectiveness of a brief, non-directive person-centred Practice. *The Person-centred Journal*, *10*, 31–38. Available at: http://adpca.org/system/files/documents/journal/5%20PCJ%2010.pdf

Feltham, C. (1995) *What is Counseling? The Promise and Problem of the Talking Therapies*. London: Sage.

Feltham, C. & Dryden, W. (2006) *Brief Counselling: A Practical Integrative Approach*, 2nd edition. New York: Open University.

Freire, E., Elliot, R. & Westwell, G. (2013) Person-centred and Experiential Psychotherapy Scale (PCEPS): Development and reliability of an adherence/competence measure for person-centred and experiential psychotherapies. *Counselling and Psychotherapy Research*, *14*(3), 220–226. doi:10.1080/14733145.2013.808682

Gibbard, I. & Hanley, T. (2008) A five-year evaluation of the effectiveness of person-centred counselling in routine clinical practice in primary care. *Counselling and Psychotherapy Research*, *8*(4), 215–222.

Maslow, A.H. (1943) A theory of human motivation. *Psychological Review*, *50*(4).

O'Hara, M. (1999) Moments of eternity: Carl Rogers and the contemporary demand for brief therapy. In Fairhurst, I. (Ed.), *Women Writing in the Person-Centred Approach* (pp. 63–77). Llangarron: PCCS Books.

Proctor, G., Cooper, M., Sanders, P. & Malcolm, B. (2006) *Politicizing the Person-centered Approach: An Agenda for Social Change*. Ross-on-Wye: PCCS Books.

Pybis, J., Saxon, D., Hill, A. & Barkham, M. (2017) The comparative effectiveness and efficiency of cognitive behaviour therapy and generic counselling in the treatment of depression: Evidence from the 2nd UK National Audit of psychological therapies. *BMC Psychiatry*, *17*, 215. Available at: https://bmcpsychiatry.biomedcentral.com/articles/10.1186/s12888-017-1370-7View

Rogers, C.R. (1957) The necessary and sufficient conditions of therapeutic personality change. *Journal of Consulting Psychology*, *21*, 95–103.

Rogers, C.R. (1959) The essence of psychotherapy: A client-centred view. In Tudor, K. (2008) *Brief Person-centred Therapies*. London: Sage.

Rogers, C.R. (2003) *Client Centred Therapy*. London: Constable.

Rogers, C.R. (2004) *On Becoming a Person*. London: Constable.

Sanders, P. (2004) *The Tribes of the Person-centred Nation: A Guide to the Schools of Therapy Associated with the Person-centred Approach*. Ross-on-Wye: PCCS Books.

Sanders, P. & Hill, A. (2014) *Counselling for Depression: A Person-centred and Experiential Approach to Practice*. London: Sage.

Stiles, W., Barkham, M., Mellor-Clark, J. & Connell, J. (2008) Effectiveness of cognitive-behavioural, person-centred, and psychodynamic therapies in UK primary-care routine practice: Replication in a larger sample. *Psychological Medicine, 38*(5), 677–688. doi:10.1017/S0033291707001511

Taft, J. (1933) The dynamics of therapy in a controlled relationship. New York: Macmillan

Thorne, B. (1999) The move towards brief therapy: Its dangers and challenges. *Counsellings. 10*(1), 7–11. In Tudor, K. (2008) *Brief Person-centred Therapies*. London: Sage.

Timulak, L. & Lietaer, G. (2001) Moments of empowerment: A qualitative analysis of positively experienced episodes in brief person-centred counselling. *Counselling and Psychotherapy Research, 1*(1), 62–73. doi:10.1080/147331401123313 85268

Tudor, K. (2008) *Brief Person-centred Therapies*. London: Sage.

Van Deurzen, E. (2012) *Existential Counselling & Psychotherapy in Practice*. London: Sage.

3

MOTIVATIONAL INTERVIEWING

SARAH PARRY

INTRODUCTION

This chapter will discuss the theoretical basis and practical implementation of motivational interviewing (MI). We will look at where MI came from, how MI is used, and what makes MI uniquely useful as a brief intervention in a range of settings. In brief:

- MI is an evidence-based approach that can be used transdiagnostically and works on the basis that there are particular 'target behaviours' that a person wishes to change.
- MI can be a particularly helpful approach when facilitating decision-making and supporting someone to consider whether they wish to make changes, and if so, how they will commit to doing so.
- MI is future-focused, change orientated, collaborative and person-centred, originally developing from Rogerian counselling.
- MI techniques can be used flexibly and interchangeably with other approaches; it is the 'Spirit' of MI that needs to be maintained.
- MI is guided by four key principles: express empathy, explore incongruities (where the person is and where they want to be), roll with resistance and support self-efficacy (Miller & Rollnick, 2002).

This chapter aims to:

- introduce MI as a flexible approach that moves at the client's pace and uses techniques interchangeably, as and when suitable

- explore the techniques that MI draws upon to be a collaborative, respectful and empowering approach for the client
- discuss how MI is a change-orientated conversation that can help in recognising potentially problematic behaviours, facilitating informed decision-making and positive behaviour change for clients who are ready.

WHAT IS THE EVIDENCE BASE FOR MOTIVATIONAL INTERVIEWING?

Motivational interviewing originates from Rogerian theory, which takes an optimistic perspective on the capabilities, agency for choice and change, and self-actualisation that humans have. Although the therapist takes a guiding and directive approach in MI, towards recognising discrepancies in values and behaviours thus encouraging change, the therapeutic relationship operates as equal and client-led. The MI therapist does not operate as an expert or look for pathology – emotional difficulties and distress are associated as a normal part of the human experience.

MI, as we know it today, was developed by Miller and Rollnick (1991) and is an attitude and way of connecting with someone in a particular way, rather than a discrete therapeutic approach. MI was originally used to support people who wished to make behaviour changes around substance use (see Garner et al., 2017), although MI has a wide range of uses, as we will explore throughout this chapter. Due to MI's background in behaviour change for very specific behaviours around addiction, there are three concepts that have underpinned its development, as illustrated in Figure 3.1.

The rapid rise in interest around using MI has more recently translated into a surge in research interest too, with two large meta-analyses indicating that MI is useful for a range

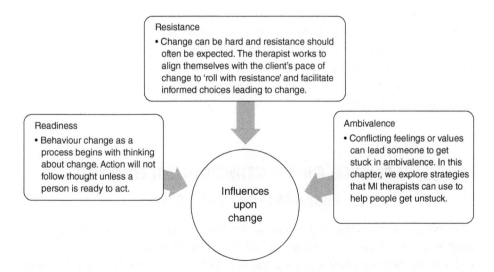

Figure 3.1   Three key influences upon change within the MI approach

of difficulties, or target behaviours (Burke, Arkowitz & Menchola, 2003; Hettema, Steele & Miller, 2005; Lundahl & Burke, 2009). Additionally, Dr Cathy Atkinson recently undertook a fascinating review with Kevin Woods (2017), exploring the theoretical stability and treatment integrity of MI, which are important factors if we are to investigate and evaluate MI work efficiently. Perhaps unsurprisingly, Cathy and Kevin found there was huge variety in how MI was practised, which makes systematic research difficult. However, this fluidity and variation also highlight the flexibility of the approach, which many practitioners are clearly utilising. MI is very much an approach used across professions, from social work (Sampson, Zayas, & Seifert, 2013) to nursing (Wu & Lin, 2009), practitioner psychology (Dean et al., 2016), physiotherapy (McGrane, Galvin, Cusack, & Stokes, 2015) and many more.

Brief forms of MI have been used to good effect in a wide variety of contexts. For example, four or fewer MI contacts (even when offered by telephone) with the aim of reducing sexual behaviours that were considered risky among HIV-positive older adults were shown to reduce target behaviours as well as depression, anxiety and stress (Lovejoy, 2012). Similarly, a four-session MI intervention for new mothers who were experiencing depression and anxiety found that new mothers who had access to an MI protocol aimed at hearing their story and accessing support services were four times more likely to seek help for emotional distress than those who did not (Holt, Milgrom, & Gemmill, 2017). Interestingly, for mothers who sought psychological support, those in the MI group were more than twice as likely to attend six or more sessions compared to the routine treatment group.

Further, employing MI as a pre-cognitive behavioural therapy intervention also appears effective for people experiencing severe generalised anxiety (Westra, Arkowitz, & Dozois, 2009), anxiety following a traumatic brain injury (Hsieh et al., 2012; Ponsford et al., 2016), and depression for young people (Hoek et al., 2011). Using brief MI as an adjunct to other approaches highlights how working with target behaviours and values prior to commencing longer-term therapy can lead to meaningful personal insights and effective outcomes. Brief MI has also been found to enhance engagement in therapy and with mental health services (Carroll et al., 2006; Dean et al., 2016; Lawrence, Fulbrook, Somerset, & Schulz, 2017).

A PRACTICAL GUIDE TO MOTIVATIONAL INTERVIEWING
FOUNDATIONS – THE 'SPIRIT' OF MI

Underlying the application of MI must be the 'Spirit' (Miller & Rollnick, 2002), as this is what sets the scene for collaboration and builds the therapeutic relationship for the conversation between client and therapist. The Spirit, or way of being with the client, conveys authentic compassion, acceptance, collaboration and respect – MI should feel like the meeting of two equals and operates on a 'non-expert' framework. The four parts of the MI Spirit are illustrated in Figure 3.2.

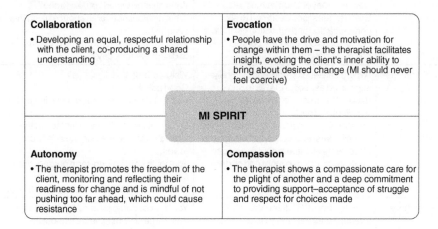

Collaboration
• Developing an equal, respectful relationship with the client, co-producing a shared understanding

Evocation
• People have the drive and motivation for change within them – the therapist facilitates insight, evoking the client's inner ability to bring about desired change (MI should never feel coercive)

MI SPIRIT

Autonomy
• The therapist promotes the freedom of the client, monitoring and reflecting their readiness for change and is mindful of not pushing too far ahead, which could cause resistance

Compassion
• The therapist shows a compassionate care for the plight of another and a deep commitment to providing support–acceptance of struggle and respect for choices made

Figure 3.2   Illustrative summary of the MI Spirit, based on Miller & Rollnick (2013) and Moyers (2014)

MOTIVATION FOR CHANGE – OARS: OPEN-ENDED QUESTIONS, AFFIRMATIONS, REFLECTIONS AND SUMMARIES

OARS are a conversational technique used within MI to begin the process of exploring the client's sense of reference to themselves, their values and the difficulty they wish to address (their target behaviour). OARS are typically used most frequently during the early stages of an intervention to elicit information and guide the conversation towards identifying the desired change, exploring barriers or costs to change, and what the benefits of change may be. Drawing on the person-centred roots of MI, attentive reflective listening and expressing empathy facilitate the OARS process, which is outlined in Table 3.1. In terms of agreeing upon a problem or target behaviour, a technique that I personally find helpful is one recommended by MI trainer Steve Berg-Smith, which includes asking the client to write down their problems or target behaviours, placing each 'target' in its own circle, in no particular pattern on the page. This process often breaks down the challenges into small achievable goals, allowing the client to choose one at a time. This level of focus can be particularly helpful for brief forms of MI. Steve Berg-Smith discusses how the circles reduce the presence of a hierarchy and offer containing bubbles/balloons for what may feel like overwhelming challenges.

Table 3.1 Overview of OARS in practice

OARS	Purpose and description	Examples
Open questions	Questions designed to encourage broader thought as well as answers – answers that are more complex than 'yes', 'no', 'maybe', 'sometimes', etc. Broader questions designed to elicit contemplation and reflection can help a person consider different perspectives and more options.	What has brought you here today? What impact does 'the problem' have on your life day-to-day? What change would you like to see? What are your concerns about making this change? What would be different if 'the problem' were to disappear for a day?
Affirmations	A more challenging and less culturally supported aspect of OARS (e.g. in the UK) but crucial for empowering the client and nurturing their sense of autonomy. These genuine and authentic compliments, appreciative reflections or statements of esteem can also inspire confidence, open thought and nurture the therapeutic relationship.	Well spotted! Good point! It sounds like you coped with that incredibly well. For you, it was really important to put their feelings first, because kindness is important to you. You could see the long-term perspective and... You managed to stay objective, even though...
Reflections	Adopted from PCT, this mode of attentive listening is used to check or convey understanding and warmth. Reflections may include a re-wording or paraphrasing of the client's accounts, establishing a shared platform of understanding before moving the conversations forwards.	You have become so used to 'the problem' that it is hard to imagine life without it. You feel as though changing the 'target behaviour' would make a big difference to some areas of your life, although it feels overwhelming when you think about where to start. 'The problem' has taken up a lot of your time and energy, you are tired by it.
Summaries	Another type of reflective listening but often longer and in more depth than a 'simple' reflection (different types of reflection discussed later). Summaries offer a checking function, alongside identifying key elements of the conversation or change talk, consolidating what has been said or shifting focus.	'The problem' has taken a lot of your time and energy, and you are understandably anxious as to how to take these first steps, but you feel it is important that you try. That sounds really important to you, can I check I understand correctly, ..., does that sound right to you? It sounds as though..., is that right? I hear that..., have I understood that properly?

TOP TIP

If it feels as though the client is 'moving away' or providing shorter and shorter answers to your questions, ask fewer questions! Get the conversation back on track by offering a thoughtful reflection or summary to show how you are listening.

Something I always try to bear in mind is that if people's difficulties were easy to solve, I would not be seeing them; they would have sorted it on their own, or with family and friends. People seek help for challenging issues when they feel stuck, so we should always be prepared for that and have strategies to hand. Within MI, strategic reflections can be a powerful way to recognise barriers to change, look at them from different perspectives and consider what options might not have been visible beforehand. Using OARS as a flexible range of tools can help keep the conversation going in a guided way to facilitate the client's awareness of underlying drivers or values, their self-awareness and enhance their confidence to achieve their ultimate goal.

Table 3.2 Examples of reflections when rolling with resistance

Strategic reflection	Examples
Client: 'I don't plan to quit drinking anytime soon!'	
Simple reflection	You don't think that quitting would work for you just now.
Amplified reflection	So your wife, children and doctor are really needlessly worrying, as you don't see drinking as a problem just now.
Double-sided reflections	You want your health and fitness to improve but you're not ready to think about quitting completely. 'Wanting two things at the same time' / 'On the one hand...'
Agreement with a twist	Yes, good point, this is bigger than just stopping drinking. It is important we bear that in mind. There's a lot going on here, besides the drinking. Drinking can affect all aspects of a person's life; it is a complicated process to think about.
Personal choice and control	You feel as though people close to you are putting a lot of pressure on you, but ultimately, this is your choice to make – your life, your body, and you are in the driving seat.
Complex reflections	It's important to you that you don't feel pushed; the challenges connected with this decision are huge! You feel as though other people's expectations are way too high just now!
Focus shift	It is not my place to tell you what to do, or even to give advice. My role is to explore options with you. You mentioned before you tend to drink more when you feel lonely; can you tell me more about that?
When there is discord in the therapeutic relationship:	
Use the 6 Rs: Recognise – Reflect – Repair – Reconnect – Reverse – Restore	
A re-balancing reflection	'I realise I'm trying to tell you what I think is right... I think this may be because... I'd like to see if we can go back and get back on track, what do you think?'

TOP TIP

Avoid the 'righting reflex' or suggesting what you think they should do. Without necessarily meaning to, we create challenges and barriers, which can mean the client moves away from our 'fixing'. Avoid 'problem-solving' language, e.g. 'Have you tried...?', 'Have you considered...?'.

LISTENING TO AND RESPONDING TO CHANGE TALK AND THE DARN CAT!

This is not an actual cat, but rather an *aide-mémoire* to highlight the stages of preparatory change talk and implementing change talk. Both of these processes (DARN and CAT) are required for meaningful and long-term change (Figure 3.3).

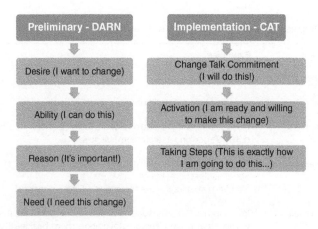

Figure 3.3 DARN CAT

When listening for change talk, there are some specific therapeutic strategies for recognising, reflecting and evoking further change talk to keep the conversation moving forwards. For example, returning to OARS, asking evocative open questions is more likely to lead to change talk than more closed questioning styles. Additionally, exploring decisional balance, weighing up the pros and cons, positives and negatives, costs and benefits of change or the status quo can help someone become unstuck in particularly complex and multifaceted circumstances. Building upon this further, asking for elaboration or examples of instances where there has been change already can elicit further change talk (e.g. 'In what ways?', 'Tell me more?', 'What does that look like?', 'When was the last time that happened?'). Changing perspectives through looking back or forwards in time can also help someone become less stuck in the present moment.

- Looking back: How can the past inform the present and future? How were things in the past better, worse or different? *'Tell me about a time before your thorough approach to cleaning became difficult for you to manage? How were things better or different?'*
- Looking forward: What would happen if the status quo remained? What would be the cost or benefit? A Solution-Focused Brief Therapy (SFBT) Miracle Question (see Chapter 4) can also be helpful here to encourage a future-orientated visualisation.

Considering extremes can also be useful. For example, in a worst-case scenario, 'What would happen if you made no changes?' And in a best-case scenario, 'What would be good about making these changes?', 'If you made the changes you have discussed, how would you know?', 'What would be different or better?'

- Considering extremes: Similarly, using rulers and scales can help someone gain some emotional distance from the 'problem'. Using numerical, word-based or pictorial scales, the therapist and client can consider how change can be observed and monitored (e.g. 'Why are you at 4 and not 3?', 'What would help you move from 4 to a 5?'). Additional questions around confidence and commitment can also be very helpful here, as a person is unlikely to make big changes if something else is more important or if they do not feel they can do it (e.g. 'How confident are you that you can make this change?', 'How committed are you to making this change?'). As confidence and commitment are so key in terms of whether the client wants to and intends to make a change in their target behaviour, it is imperative that their thoughts, perspectives of their abilities and current commitment are explored.

WHAT DOES THE CLIENT THINK?

- Do I think it is important to make a change?
- Am I confident I can make change?
- Am I committed to make change?

As a training option:

- 0–10, with zero being the lowest, how important is it to you to learn more about MI today?
- How confident are you that you can learn more about MI and have a go at it today?
- How committed are you to learn and have a go?
  - *Why score X not Y?*
  - *What would you need to move from X to Y?*
  - *How might life be different?*
  - *What could increase your confidence?*

Another important consideration within MI is to explore a person's core values. There are several values-based questionnaires freely available online, especially through Acceptance and Commitment Therapy resource centres. For clients who may be more aware of their values system, you can also ask what a person's guiding values are, what they want from life, and how their current actions align with these values. For example, if someone wants to give up smoking as a target behaviour and one of their core values is looking after their overall health, this highlights a dissonance that can be recognised and addressed. One technique in this instance, if the therapeutic alliance is strong enough, is to play devil's advocate. For a moment, playfully take the side of the target behaviour and question whether it is so important, so valued and so needed that it is not worth giving up or challenging.

When exploring change talk and maintaining a forward focus, try to follow these guideposts to keep you on track:

- Reinforce change – keep the client on their chosen course (use the bubble list)
- Stay on the client's path, avoid the righting reflex
- Be alert – don't go too fast and fall into advice giving or the righting reflex
- Keep in the Spirit and partnership
- The client is much more likely to shift to resistance if resistance talk is not heard by the therapist and responded to. The illustration in Figure 3.4 demonstrates how transitional summaries can be used to facilitate or initiate change talk in the face of sustain talk.

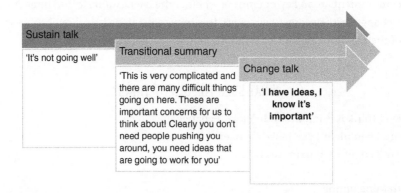

Figure 3.4   Transitional summaries

Knowing when the client is ready to act on change talk and plan for change can be a tricky judgement to make. However, there are some signs you can look out for, which should signal you can begin to develop an action plan for change with the client. For example, a client who usually focuses on the past or present may begin to discuss life in the future after changes are made. The client may seek advice or ask questions about making particular changes, indicating that they are contemplating change (see Prochaska & DiClemente's transtheoretical stages of change model (Prochaska & DiClemente, 1983)), or try out new strategies or techniques in-between sessions and feedback to you. These are all signs you can begin a collaborative action plan for change with the client, which may resemble that in Table 3.3.

Table 3.3   Action plan for change process

Component	Process
Summary	• What are the client's reasons for change that they have identified or implied?
	• Can a transitional summary be employed, to recognise any anxieties or remaining ambivalence, while recognising and affirming the client's commitment to and confidence in the identified change?

Component	Process
Focused questions	• OARS – open questions: 'Where could you go from here?', 'What do you think are the next steps?' – affirm, reflect, summarise.
Psychoeducation within the Spirit	• ONLY when invited or permitted, some relevant psychoeducation, signposting, information about what others find helpful or even advice based on the evidence base and/or theory can be offered to inform the client's plan.
The plan	• Explore options for change; weigh them up against one another and the status quo – What is the first goal? What is the priority? • OARS – Why this goal? – affirm, reflect, summarise. • Commitment – Is this definitely what they want to do? What personal value is this commitment connecting with? Why is it personally meaningful to them? – affirm, reflect, summarise. • Confidence – Do they feel they can do it? Who could help? How? When? What personal resources do they have? What change have they already initiated by themselves? – affirm, reflect, summarise. • CHANGE PLAN – What are the steps? How will they be achieved? – affirm, reflect, summarise. • How will the client know change has occurred? Will they let you know? Why?

TOP TIP

Engaging with therapy should be an informed choice; MI can be very useful when helping someone arrive at an informed choice after considering their stage of readiness, motivation, values and barriers. Making this choice can, on its own, be very therapeutic and empowering.

STORIES FROM PRACTICE

Readiness for therapy and informed decision-making

June was in her early 50s when she was re-referred to the local community mental health team. She was always impeccably dressed, with manicured nails and styled hair. She lived with her husband and spent a great deal of her time with her show dogs and friends, who also had dogs. June had contact with the mental health team every two to three years, and was usually referred around Christmas time. This pattern had lasted over ten years and included two hospital admissions over the last four years. From reading through June's notes and speaking with other members of the team who had worked with her through the years, there were indications that June would go for periods of time seeming well, although she would also have phases during the winter of extreme low mood. During these phases, June would largely stay in bed, struggle with communication and self-care, couldn't walk her dogs and her husband would request an increase in her lithium dose and psychological support for her. During the last request from her husband for psychology input, he had explained that June had been mentioning her father, although he couldn't make out what she had been trying to say and June had not wanted to discuss this since.

When I met with June initially, it was early spring as she had been waiting for a psychology appointment for some months. June told me she sometimes found the Christmas holidays

(Continued)

difficult, although was 'fine the rest of the time' and 'certainly didn't need therapy'. June explained that people 'of her generation didn't do therapy' and had 'other ways to cope'. I asked June how she coped with difficult things and she replied that she 'just didn't think about them'. By this point, I was mindful that June did not want to engage in psychological therapy and that, as such, this might be our last meeting. However, perhaps just wishing to change the subject and knowing I was new to the service, June asked how I was settling in. I replied and then asked June a few open questions about her contact with the service in the past, such as what had been helpful and who she had enjoyed spending time with.

I reflected to June that she seemed to have a good relationship with one of the mental health nurses, who also spoke warmly of June, and asked what she knew about psychological therapy. June replied, 'I know it's about talking about the past, I don't like thinking about the past', to which I reflected, 'Thinking about things that have happened in the past is difficult, and it sounds as though you have a very fun and fulfilling life now that you enjoy, so you don't feel as though therapy would be helpful, is that right?' June agreed and then told me more about her dogs and friends, showing me some pictures on her phone and explained that she enjoyed keeping busy and focusing on the here and now. June then paused and said that she knew she had her 'struggles', but that she coped most of the time and didn't want to dig up the past. Given that June had volunteered some information about her struggles, I asked some simple open questions about how keeping busy seemed to help and what the impact of her struggles could be day-to-day.

June explained that she worried sometimes about 'feeling low', taking the lithium that could make her hands shake, and that she missed out on things she enjoyed when she was struggling, but she didn't think therapy was for her. I explained that engaging in any thera-peutic work had to be June's choice and reflected that she had clearly considered her options and knew what was best for her. At this point, June asked if therapy always needed to be about the past. Invited to provide some further information and with change talk observed, I explained to June that therapeutic support could also be about coping in the moment and planning. June thanked me for the information and asked if she could have some 'thinking time' to consider her options. I reaffirmed that engaging in a therapeutic process would need to be June's decision and that the service could leave a two-week window for her to decide.

After a few days, June contacted the mental health nurse she knew well and asked to set up four initial psychology sessions, highlighting that she wanted to focus on 'coping strategies for the here and now'. In this instance, MI facilitated an informed choice and the client's autonomy to request a particular approach. The subsequent four sessions were informed largely by CBT, with identified goals around monitoring and challenging anxious thoughts and avoidant behav-iours. However, through incorporating OARS into therapeutic conversations and maintaining the Spirit of MI, June appeared to feel more in control and in a position to resolve the ambiv-alence between wanting to 'feel more like herself' and less anxious, in contrast to her fears around 'opening up old wounds'. During our fourth and final planned session, again employing OARS, we had a conversation around the potential costs and benefits of undertaking further therapy. June decided she would like another eight sessions, exploring her feelings in relation to times when she was unwell. This work took the form of PCT, although with the MI Spirit embed-ded in the relationship and conversations employing MI techniques for additional structure. This process led June to a point where she could comfortably and actively engage in a style of therapy she considered helpful. With additional awareness, coping strategies and organised channels through which she could ask for help when she felt 'the struggles' appearing, June's overall health improved and she did not have further emergency admissions to the team.

Pacing and Making Changes

Stuart was in his mid-40s when he was referred to the psychology department of a specialist pain clinic. Stuart had persistent neuropathic pain, which led to flare-ups and periods of intense pain and discomfort. Stuart also worked full-time as an academic and described himself as 'ambitious', 'a perfectionist', 'work-hard, play-hard type'. Stuart was used to pushing himself at work, making the most of late nights, making sacrifices, and employed two key coping strategies: 'do more', 'work harder'. However, over the previous three years, Stuart had experienced a significant increase in his pain, which caused him a great deal of stress, which he recognised increased the likelihood of tension and flare-ups. True to form, Stuart had engaged fully in a pain management course and worked hard to keep his physical fitness high, although he had not seen an improvement.

Stuart came to psychology with a desire for more coping strategies and techniques he could try. Using open questions, I asked Stuart about what he had tried so far, what impact he thought these strategies had had, and what he wanted in the future. Affirmations were particularly important for Stuart at the time as he felt he had 'tried everything' and was feeling very anxious about his future. Through a series of reflections (largely personal control and complex reflections), we explored Stuart's values system that was driving his 'do more', 'try harder', 'keep pushing' strategies. One of Stuart's options was to actively do less, to rest, and accept that his body was signalling to him to slow down a little. This was a difficult action for Stuart to realistically consider, as this would require moving away from striving and actively challenged how he saw himself. However, Stuart quickly initiated change talk ('I want...', 'I'm just worried that...', 'I'm tired of...', 'I'd like to be able to...') and identified that his core values were more aligned to keeping well and having energy for relationships and his career, rather than to continuing to push himself with little visible benefit to his health. Therefore, some careful considerations using OARS were employed around the target behaviour (pushing himself too hard) and change (see Figures 3.5 and 3.6).

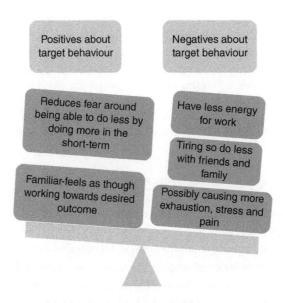

Figure 3.5   Weighing up positives and negatives around change

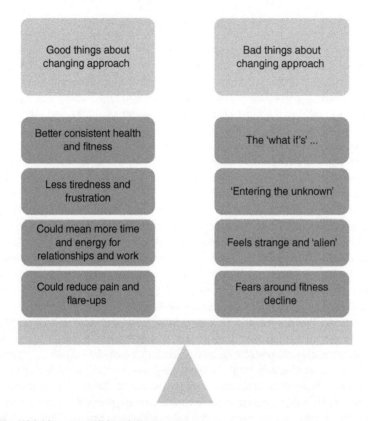

Figure 3.6 Weighing up possible outcomes

Following these analyses, we considered confidence and commitment scales and how Stuart could be supported as he tried a new approach. This then led to the development of a change plan, with integrated regular review meetings with the psychologist and physiotherapist to monitor his emotional and physical health. Stuart also began attending a mindfulness group, which met his needs in terms of mindful awareness of his body's signals as well as soothing his mind and body, while also helping him feel as though he was still actively managing his condition through activity. The results were positive and this led to a new management plan for Stuart's pain that he could self-manage and feel positive about.

CONCLUSION

- MI is a collaborative talking therapy between two equals that is rooted in humanism but is structured and guided.
- MI can only truly operate when the Spirit of MI becomes a way of being in the therapeutic space, involving collaboration, autonomy, evocation and compassion.
- Attentive and reflective listening can move the process of change forward, with skilfully crafted questions based on the language of the client.

- MI is powerful, dynamic and often fast-paced, making it a great option for a brief therapeutic intervention for people with clear and identified goals around behaviour change.

DISCUSSION QUESTIONS
---

1. What may attract therapists and clients to a MI approach? Would therapists and clients be attracted by the same features of MI?
2. What may be some of the barriers to utilising MI in statutory services, compared to private practice?
3. How might the flexibility of MI in practice act as a barrier to the systematic investigation of the efficacy of MI for research purposes?
4. Is MI still MI if practitioners struggle to accept and implement 'the Spirit'?

KEY TERMS

Ambivalence Conflicting feelings about change – wanting two things at the same time – which can stall the process of change.

Change talk Linguistic signals that the client is contemplating change, which may include problem recognition statements, expressing concern about the status quo, expressions of desire (e.g. 'I want to stop...', 'I want to start...') or optimism (e.g. 'I know this is possible for me').

Reflective listening A listening style from PCT, through which the therapist demonstrates careful and attuned listening through accurate summaries to check understanding (see Chapter 2 for further description and examples).

FURTHER READING

- Rollick, S., Miller, W. R., & Moyers, T. B. (Eds). (2012). *Applications of Motivational Interviewing*. New York: Guilford Press. A fantastic 'how to' of MI, with examples and discussion.
- Zuckoff, S. (2015). *Finding Your Way to Change: How the Power of Motivational Interviewing Can Reveal What You Want and Help You Get There*. New York: Guilford Press. ISBN 9781462520404. A book designed to help guide you through self-directed MI to overcome challenges and find resolutions.
- Naar, S., & Suarez, M. (2010). *Motivational Interviewing with Adolescents and Young Adults*. New York: Guilford Press. ISBN-10: 1609180623. A comprehensive practitioner guide with examples, discussions and do's and don'ts of using MI with young people.
- MI Resources – Motivational Interviewing Network of Trainers: www.motivationalinter viewing.org/motivational-interviewing-resources
- Motivational Interviewing, Psychology Tools: https://psychologytools.com/technique-motivational-interviewing.html
- Free MI Resources – Motivational Interviewing: http://miinlondon.org/motivational-inter viewing-free-resources
- Motivational Interviewing Resources – Mi-CCSI: www.miccsi.org/motivational-interview ing-resources

- We have recently set up a new network for people interested in MI that is based in Greater Manchester but open to all. Please follow us on Twitter for updates @GM_MI_Network or visit our new website at www.mmin.co.uk

REFERENCES

Atkinson, C., & Woods, K. (2017). Establishing theoretical stability and treatment integrity for motivational interviewing. *Behavioural and Cognitive Psychotherapy, 45*(4), 337–350. doi:10.1017/S1352465817000145

Burke, B. L., Arkowitz, H., & Menchola, M. (2003). The efficacy of motivational interviewing: A meta-analysis of controlled clinical trials. *Journal of Consulting and Clinical Psychology, 71*, 843–861.

Carroll, K. M., Ball, S. A., Nich, C., Martino, S., Frankforter, T. L., Farentinos, C., Kunkel, L. E., Mikulich-Gilbertson, S. K., Morgenstern, J., Obert, J. L., & Polcin, D. (2006). Motivational interviewing to improve treatment engagement and outcome in individuals seeking treatment for substance abuse: A multisite effectiveness study. *Drug and Alcohol Dependence, 81*(3), 301–312. doi:10.1016/j.drugalcdep.2005.08.002

Dean, S., Britt, E., Bell, E., Stanley, J., & Collings, S. (2016). Motivational interviewing to enhance adolescent mental health treatment engagement: A randomized clinical trial. *Psychological Medicine, 46*(9), 1961–1969. doi:10.1017/S0033291716000568

Garner, B. R., Gotham, H. J., Tueller, S. J., Ball, E. L., Kaiser, D., Stilen, P., Speck, K., Vandersloot, D., Rieckmann, T. R., Chaple, M., Martin, E. G., & Martino, S. (2017). Testing the effectiveness of a motivational interviewing-based brief intervention for substance use as an adjunct to usual care in community-based AIDS service organizations: Study protocol for a multisite randomized controlled trial. *Addiction Science & Clinical Practice, 12*(1), 1–15.

Hettema, J., Steele, J., & Miller, W. R. (2005). Motivational interviewing. *Annual Review of Clinical Psychology, 1*, 91–111.

Hoek, W., Marko, M., Fogel, J., Schuurmans, J., Gladstone, T., Bradford, N., ... Van Voorhees, B. W. (2011). Randomized controlled trial of primary care physician motivational interviewing versus brief advice to engage adolescents with an internet-based depression prevention intervention: 6-month outcomes and predictors of improvement. *Translational Research, 158*(6), 315–325. doi:10.1016/j.trsl.2011.07.006

Holt, C., Milgrom, J., & Gemmill, A. W. (2017). Improving help-seeking for postnatal depression and anxiety: A cluster randomised controlled trial of motivational interviewing. *Archives of Women's Mental Health, 20*(6), 791–801. doi:10.1007/s00737-017-0767-0

Hsieh, M., Ponsford, J., Wong, D., Schönberger, M., McKay, A., & Haines, K. (2012). Development of a motivational interviewing programme as a prelude to CBT for anxiety following traumatic brain injury. *Neuropsychological Rehabilitation, 22*(4), 563. doi.org/10.1080/09602011.2012.676284

Lawrence, P., Fulbrook, P., Somerset, S., & Schulz, P. (2017). Motivational interviewing to enhance treatment attendance in mental health settings: A systematic review and meta-analysis. *Journal of Psychiatric and Mental Health Nursing*, *24*(9–10), 699–718. doi:10.1111/jpm.12420

Lovejoy, T. I. (2012). Telephone-delivered motivational interviewing targeting sexual risk behavior reduces depression, anxiety, and stress in HIV-positive older adults. *Annals of Behavioral Medicine*, *44*(3), 416–421. doi:10.1007/s12160-012-9401-6

Lundahl, B., & Burke, B. L. (2009). The effectiveness and applicability of motivational interviewing: A practice-friendly review of four meta-analyses. *Journal of Clinical Psychology*, *65*: 1232–1245. doi:10.1002/jclp.20638

McGrane, N., Galvin, R., Cusack, T., & Stokes, E. (2015). Addition of motivational interventions to exercise and traditional physiotherapy: A review and meta-analysis. *Physiotherapy*, *101*(1), 1–12. doi:10.1016/j.physio.2014.04.009

Miller, W. R., & Rollnick, S. (1991). *Motivational interviewing: Preparing people to change addictive behavior*. London, New York: Guilford Press.

Miller, W. R., & Rollnick, S. (2002). *Motivational interviewing: Preparing people for change* (2nd ed.). London, New York: Guilford Press.

Miller, W. R., & Rollnick, S. (2013). *Motivational interviewing: Helping people change* (3rd ed.). New York: Guilford Publications.

Moyers, T. B. (2014). The relationship in motivational interviewing. *Psychotherapy*, *51*(3), 358–363.

Ponsford, J., Lee, N. K., Wong, D., McKay, A., Haines, K., Alway, Y., Downing, M., Furtado, C., & O'Donnell, M. L. (2016). Efficacy of motivational interviewing and cognitive behavioral therapy for anxiety and depression symptoms following traumatic brain injury. *Psychological Medicine*, *46*(5), 1079.

Prochaska, J. O., & DiClemente, C. C. (1983). Stages and processes of self-change of smoking: Toward an integrative model of change. *Journal of Consulting and Clinical Psychology*, *51*(3), 390–395.

Sampson, M., Zayas, L. H., & Seifert, S. B. (2013). Treatment engagement using motivational interviewing for low-income, ethnically diverse mothers with postpartum depression. *Clinical Social Work Journal*, *41*(4), 387–394. doi:10.1007/s10615-012-0422-1

Westra, H. A., Arkowitz, H., & Dozois, D. J. A. (2009). Adding a motivational interviewing pretreatment to cognitive behavioral therapy for generalized anxiety disorder: A preliminary randomized controlled trial. *Journal of Anxiety Disorders*, *23*(8), 1106–1117. doi:10.1016/j.janxdis.2009.07.014

Wu, C., & Lin, C. (2009). The application of motivational interviewing in nursing practice. *Hu Li Za Zhi/The Journal of Nursing*, *56*(2), 89.

4

SOLUTION-FOCUSED BRIEF THERAPY
PANORAIA ANDRIOPOULOU AND SARAH PARRY

INTRODUCTION

Problem talk creates problems, Solution talk creates solutions.

(Steve de Shazer, cited in Berg & Szabó, 2005, p. 1)

Solution-Focused Brief Therapy (SFBT) is a brief, future and solution-orientated model, which explores 'what works' rather than problems or complaints. Unlike other approaches, the focus of SFBT is on those occasions where the symptom or the problem does *not* occur. Therefore, the therapist's aim is to identify those 'exceptions' and collaboratively investigate with the client what they *do* differently or what *is* different in general when the problem is absent. The ultimate goal of SFBT is to induce positive change by broadening and building on those 'exceptions', as, according to the model, even minor positive changes can initiate and establish a positive spiral of continuing change. This chapter offers an overview of the approach and its interventions.

Specifically, this chapter will discuss:

- The history and background of Solution-Focused Brief Therapy
- The nature of the therapeutic relationship in Solution-Focused Brief Therapy
- The course of Solution-Focused Brief Therapy and its interventions
- An evaluation of the Solution-Focused Model

The chapter aims to:

- familiarise the reader with the SFBT approach and how it conceptualises clients' strengths and difficulties
- provide a clear, step-by-step account of how the model operates in practice
- familiarise the reader with the main techniques of the approach and how these are applied.

THEORETICAL INTRODUCTION TO SFBT

Solution-Focused Brief Therapy has its roots in humanism (see Chapter 3), Systemic Family Therapy and the early work of the Palo Alto Group and Mental Research Institute (MRI) therapists (see Chapter 5 for a more detailed account of the Palo Alto model). SFBT was originally developed at the Brief Family Therapy Centre in Milwaukee by Insoo Kim Berg, Steve de Shazer and their colleagues (de Shazer, 1985; de Schazer, Dolan, Korman, Trepper, McCollum, & Berg, 2007). Similarly to MRI therapists, solution-focused therapists were not concerned with helping the client to gain insight about their problems and they did not explore cognitions, feelings or other intrapersonal processes as such. However, while MRI therapists were interested in both the clients' problems and attempted solutions, the focus of SFBT shifted from problems to solutions. The assessment phase changed and became shorter as the therapist concentrated more on the solutions instead of exploring the clients' problems in depth. Consequently, SFBT therapists helped their clients develop new solutions, or build on the ones that were already working, rather than helping them to solve problems or abandon problematic attempted solutions. The instances when the problem was not present became the focal point and clients were encouraged to describe what was different when the problem was absent. Those instances of success became known as 'exceptions' and were considered the beginning of the solution.

The model adopts an optimistic and collaborative approach, assuming that human beings are inherently motivated to reach their full potential and therefore capable of solving their own problems. Therefore, clients are considered 'experts' of their own lives and this notion is well illustrated in de Shazer's (1985, p. 6) claim that the key to brief therapy is to 'utilise what the client brings with him to meet his needs in such a way that the client can make a satisfactory life for himself'. In other words, it is the client who produces the solutions to their problems.

The model is brief, goal-directed and future-orientated. De Shazer and his colleagues believed, based on observations and relevant literature (e.g. Gurman, 1981), that clients across the board would not stay in therapy for more than 6–10 sessions. Therefore, attempting to gain a deeper understanding of how problems developed or how they were maintained was neither relevant nor necessary for change to occur and could lead to unnecessarily long treatments.

The model was pragmatically and progressively developed. Through observing a large number of sessions over the course of many years, the model's founders noted all the questions that led clients to progress and adopt successful solutions. The pertinent and successful questions formed the basis of the treatment protocol (de Shazer et al., 2007). Theoretically, SFBT embraces the humanistic and social constructionism principles by emphasising the importance of the client's own construction of reality. It is therefore considered a non-normative, non-pathologising approach. Accordingly, the problems people encounter are considered a part of the typical human experience, rather than an 'illness'. In most cases, people manage to solve their problems successfully by finding effective solutions. There are times, however, when these past solutions are not as effective anymore and clients struggle to come up with new ones. The role of the SFBT therapist is to assist the client to overcome these obstacles and find new ways of coping towards a point of fulfilment.

EVALUATION AND EFFECTIVENESS OF SFBT

There are a number of systematic reviews (e.g. Gingerich & Peterson, 2013; Franklin, Zhang, Froerer, & Johnson, 2017) and meta-analyses (e.g. Kim, 2008; Zhang, Franklin, Currin-McCulloch, Park, & Kim, 2018) supporting the effectiveness of SFBT. More specifically, SFBT has been found effective for a number of problems, such as depression and anxiety (Maljanen, Härkänen, Virtala, Lindfors, Tillman, & Knekt, 2014), behavioural difficulties in school settings (Kim & Franklin, 2009) and substance use difficulties (Smock, Trepper, Wetchler, McCollum, Ray, & Pierce, 2008). SFBT is considered an evidence-based, high-intensity psychosocial intervention and is recommended by the National Institute for Health and Care Excellence (NICE) for the treatment of depression in adults (NICE, CG90, 2009a), for depression with a chronic physical problem (NICE, CG91, 2009b) and in the care of adults with cancer (NICE, 2004).

THE BASIC TENETS OF SFBT

The basic tenets of SFBT (based on de Shazer et al., 2007) are:

1. *If it ain't broke, don't fix it.* SFBT therapists will terminate therapy when problems have been resolved and will not encourage therapy for reasons of personal growth or of gaining a deeper insight. According to the SFBT line of thinking, if there is no problem, then there should be no therapy.
2. *Once you know what works, do more of it.* The client is encouraged to continue using solutions or strategies that have been proven effective in the past and expand on them. The quality of the solutions is not important for the therapist as long as those solutions are successful. Part of the treatment, therefore, focuses on identifying those periods in the past when the client was successful in dealing with the problem and reinforcing the use of tried-and-tested solutions.
3. *If it doesn't work, don't do it again. Do something different.* If a solution to a problem does not work, then it is not the right solution. The therapist will assess those

solutions that have already been employed by the client to solve the problem but have been unsuccessful, to avoid wasting therapy time by testing solutions the client has already attempted. Similarly, if the client does not complete a task that has been suggested by the therapist, then the task is abandoned as it is considered unsuitable for the particular client.

4. *Small steps can lead to big changes.* The assumption here is that even a minimal change can bring about a series of changes by creating a positive spiral. Even small successes can be empowering for the client, helping them attempt more changes and take further steps towards achieving their goals.

5. *The solution is not necessarily related to the problem.* Identifying the cause of the problem is not important for a solution to be found. Unlike other models of therapy, which focus on insight and identification of the root of the problem, SFBT posits that it is counterproductive to spend time identifying the origins of the problem when you can invest this time in finding a solution. In other words, problem analysis does not necessarily lead to successful solutions. For this reason, the therapist and the client spend little, if any, time on analysing symptoms or difficulties, focusing instead on future goals.

6. *The language for solution development is different from that needed to describe a problem.* SFBT therapists employ a 'language of change'. Namely, the language is optimistic, motivating and future-orientated as opposed to the negative language of problems. The use of positive language also facilitates the reconstruction of the meaning of problems, giving the client the message that problems are transient and part of the normal human experience. Clients are encouraged to believe that positive change is possible and within their control.

7. *No problem happens all the time; there are always exceptions that can be utilised.* The therapist's role is to bring to light those instances when the problem is not present and identify the circumstances under which this is happening. These exceptions are then used to initiate small changes.

8. *The future is both created and negotiable.* According to this principle, people are the architects of their own future and destiny. Unlike other therapeutic approaches where the client's behaviour is considered to be governed by the negative experiences of the past, the SFBT model assumes a humanistic perspective and posits that human beings have an innate ability to strive towards self-actualisation, and the capacity to solve their own problems.

TOP TIP

Focus on solutions rather than problems. The SFBT model focuses on solution-building rather than problem-solving, encouraging a future-focused orientation, optimism and hopefulness.

ASSUMPTIONS ABOUT CLIENTS AND THE THERAPEUTIC RELATIONSHIP

SFBT is a collaborative approach and SFBT therapists adopt a 'not knowing', 'non-pathologising' stance. Therapists abandon the role of the expert and consequently avoid the use of 'expert language' or diagnoses. This approach facilitates an egalitarian and equal relationship (de Shazer et al., 2007), within which the clients' feelings are acknowledged and validated, while both therapist and client remain positive and optimistic. The therapist is therefore experienced as an encouraging and supportive companion in the client's journey towards change.

A PRACTICAL GUIDE TO SFBT

THE COURSE OF THERAPY

PRE-SESSION CHANGE

According to SFBT therapists, change starts at the time of the appointment making (Weiner-Davis, de Shazer, & Gingerich, 1987). So, one common question early in the first session is whether the client has noticed any changes or improvements in their situation already. The answer to the question will allow the therapist to focus on change from the very beginning of the therapy. The follow-up questions (e.g. 'What were these changes?', 'What have you done that brought about these changes?') will start the process of 'solution-talk' and exceptions, and will build the client's confidence by getting them to realise their strengths and capabilities.

ESTABLISHING SOLUTION-FOCUSED GOALS

As in other approaches, goals need to follow the SMART system (Latham & Locke, 2002) in the sense that they need to be specific, measurable, achievable, relevant and time-bound. Additionally, the goals have to be solution-focused rather than problem-aversive. So, for example, 'be relaxed' instead of 'experience less anxiety'.

IDENTIFYING PAST SUCCESSES AND EXCEPTIONS

The therapist will ask questions to investigate whether the client has experienced the same or a similar problem in the past and how they have dealt with it. This is a useful way for the therapist to identify strategies that have been effective in the past and assess the client's competences. In a similar way, the therapist will explore whether there have been times when the problem was absent, or less intense, even though the situations would favour its appearance. Questioning around those exceptions will again allow the therapist to become aware of the client's qualities and the resources they draw on to handle difficult situations.

DESIGNING INTERVENTIONS AND ASSIGNING TASKS WITH AN AIM TO AMPLIFY EXCEPTIONS AND INITIATE CHANGE

The therapist will work with the client to design homework assignments or experiments that will follow on from the session and will allow them to head towards a desirable goal. In many cases, these tasks will involve amplification of the exceptions, where the client has to recognise what has helped them deal with the problem in the past and build upon successful coping strategies. The client is actively engaged in the design of the experiments to ensure that these are relevant and that the client will actually do them. SFBT therapists will easily abandon a task if the client does not complete it and will consider it an unsuccessful task rather than jump to conclusions about the client's resistance.

EVALUATING THE EFFECTIVENESS OF TASKS AND IDENTIFYING POSITIVE CHANGES

The therapist and client will evaluate what is working and what is not. The client will be encouraged to continue with successful tasks that bring about positive changes whereas tasks that do not work will be abandoned and replaced by different ones.

ASSESSING TREATMENT OUTCOMES AND STABILISING GAINS

This is the stage in therapy where the gains are evaluated and compared against the initial list of goals. If the client has reached the goals set at the beginning of the therapy, then the possibility of termination is discussed and the client is encouraged to stay focused on the positive changes achieved, rather than regressing to previous behaviours. It is also possible that the client decides that they want to work on new problems and then new goals are negotiated.

TERMINATION

Termination in therapy takes place when the client feels that they have reached their goals and is satisfied with the progress they have made. Clients are also reminded that they are welcome to contact the therapist in the future, if necessary.

TECHNIQUES

THE MIRACLE QUESTION

This technique can be considered one of the major contributions of the model and it is utilised by therapists of many approaches. It is the successor of Ericson's 'crystal ball technique' (see de Shazer, 1978), where clients under hypnosis were encouraged to imagine their lives as they wanted them to be without their current problems and describe in detail the steps in the resolution of those problems. This technique is particularly useful for clients who find it difficult to elucidate specific goals and it helps define potential solutions, taking the focus off the problem (de Shazer, 1988).

The following example comes from de Shazer's (1988) version of the miracle question, although the phrasing of the question may vary depending upon the shared language developed throughout the therapeutic process.

> Suppose that one night, while you are asleep, there is a miracle and the problem that brought you here is solved. However, because you are asleep, you don't know that the miracle has already happened. When you wake up in the morning, what will be different that will tell you that the miracle has taken place? What else?

Miracle question follow-up questions might include the following:

- What difference would you (and others) notice?
- What are the first things you would notice?
- Has any of this ever happened before?
- What would need to happen to do this?
- What else?

TOP TIP

Don't create new problems. Allow the client to outline their own problems and decide on the goals they want to work towards. The role of the therapist is not to help the client identify new problems, but to work with whatever the client brings to therapy.

SCALING QUESTIONS

Scaling questions allow the client to evaluate on a rating scale, most usually from zero to 10, their goals, feelings, thoughts and successes. It is a particularly useful technique as they allow the therapist to assess progress from session to session, especially with clients who lean towards a black-or-white thinking style and struggle to recognise small changes. It is important to recognise when and how the scale goes up, and to compliment the client on their achievements, no matter how small these are. Scaling questions can also be used to assess the client's motivation to change. So consider, for example, the following question: 'On a scale of zero to 10, where zero means you are completely demotivated and 10 means you are completely motivated to reach your goals, where would you place yourself now?'

Follow-up questions could include the following (Sharry, 2007):

- Can you tell me how you know you are there and not there?
- What things have you done already that got you to this point?
- What do you think will move you one step further?
- How would you know you have made that step?

- Who would be the first person to notice that you had moved one point on?
- What would they notice about you?
- What would that mean to you?

COPING QUESTIONS

Coping questions allow the clients to focus on their strengths and on examples of having successfully coped with problems in the past rather than on failures. In this way, clients are able to recognise their effective coping mechanisms and feel optimistic about the future. Examples of coping questions might include the following: 'How have you managed to cope so well given the circumstances?', 'How have you managed to prevent things from getting worse?', 'What do you think are the qualities you have that keep you going?' (de Shazer et al., 2007; Davis & Osborn, 2013).

COMPLIMENTS AND ENCOURAGEMENT

SFBT therapists will guide their clients through questioning to describe what they did well and they will compliment them on their accomplishments. Compliments enhance the client's self-esteem and increase their motivation for change. They are also useful as they strengthen the therapeutic relationship as the therapist appears as somebody who cares and understands (Berg & Dolan, 2001). Finally, they allow the therapist to punctuate what the client has done well and should continue doing (de Shazer et al., 2007).

TOP TIP

Use optimistic and future-orientated language that focuses on change and success.

STORIES FROM PRACTICE

Jan-Scaling up the garden path

Jan was a woman in her late-50s who was accessing a community mental health clinic for anxiety and depression, following a series of operations that had involved a long convalescence period. Jan reported hypervigilance around her physical health and experienced related anxiety, in addition to a fear of over-exertion that prevented her from going out to see friends and maintaining her garden, which she had been fond of doing before her surgeries. When Jan came to clinic, she said she wanted to 'feel more like herself', which she said would be helped initially by being able to tend her garden again. Through a series of coping questions to ascertain what changes Jan had already made, it became clear that Jan had managed to move back upstairs to her bedroom, rather than sleeping in the lounge, and that she would

(Continued)

stand by her back door, looking at the garden, which had become overgrown. Jan described many self-critical thoughts about how she 'should be doing more' and worries she held about what her neighbours would think about 'the state of the garden … and me'.

Some careful time was spent acknowledging her worries and hearing about the series of surgeries that had spanned a 12-month period. Then, a scale began to emerge depicting the progresses Jan had already made in terms of her recovery and self-care. These scaling conversations led to the development of a pictorial scale, rather than a numerical scale, to illustrate Jan's desired goal to begin gardening again. Recognising the progress Jan had already made, the scale began in her bedroom and continued down the garden, ending at her shed where she kept her gardening tools and where she used to sit to enjoy her garden. Jan described herself as a visual person, so a visual representation of her goal and steps towards it seemed appropriate.

A common concern among therapists new to SFBT approaches is whether the miracle question can be construed as a little patronising by some clients. One way to navigate this with visual thinkers is to contextualise the miracle question within a metaphor–in Jan's case, this was her garden. An adapted version of the miracle question, in which Jan was pain-free and without worry for her future health, was asked. Jan described that she would know a miracle had happened because her house and garden would be 'in the order they used to be in'. Jan said she would be sitting in the sunshine outside her garden shed with a cup of tea, enjoying looking at her flowerbeds and anticipating what areas she would need to focus on next, joking that 'a gardener's work is never done'. She continued to say her neighbours would compliment her on her garden and that she would feel comfortable inviting friends and neighbours in as she wouldn't feel embarrassed. Jan recognised that although gardening gave her a sense of purpose and was an activity she enjoyed, it was the enjoyment of the garden, by herself and with her visitors, that she was really missing. When asked if Jan had ever seen the garden overgrown before, she explained that there had been so much work to do when she bought the house some years before that she had briefly hired some gardeners to help.

We returned to the scale to look at what the steps could be to get from the back door to the garden shed. Jan said that, as she still could not lift heavy loads, the first step would be to ask a gardener to help with the garden for a short period, just until she was able to take over. Jan also added a step that, with a little help, she could plant up some pots by the back door, to enjoy the garden closer to the house while her recovery continued. The scale was used to evidence the progress she was making, as Jan could gradually do more and more. A component of this section of the work was to recognise Jan's high standards for herself and to readjust her expectations to align with her recovery. Over the following weeks, Jan became more confident in her physical abilities as she began to do a little more in her home and garden. She started to invite her friends over and spent longer on the phone to her sister, which she reported was easier as she had more to tell her. As Jan's physical recovery continued and she spent more time connected to important people in her life, as well as getting back to her garden, she reported worrying less and feeling more positive. Jan had six sessions of SFBT over a three-month period.

Gordon–Going to the wedding

Gordon was in his late 40s and had undergone a number of abdominal surgeries, which had resulted in a great deal of persistent pain and the fitting of a colostomy bag. Gordon had experienced a traumatic incident some months before when the bag came loose in a shop, which had resulted in Gordon not wishing to go out in public whenever possible. After working with Gordon therapeutically for a number of weeks around his self-esteem and health-related anxiety, and liaising with his medical team around ongoing appointments, Gordon brought a specific goal to therapy, which we explored using a SFBT approach specifically. Gordon's niece was getting married and he had been invited to the wedding. Gordon explained how he desperately wanted to go, although he was completely overwhelmed with anxiety and described vividly how he had imaged all kinds of scenarios in relation to his physical health and the bag in particular.

Emotionally, Gordon said he couldn't imagine how he could go. Cue the miracle question, although again in this case it was rephrased: 'Imagine you've already been, what did you see?' Phrasing the question to evoke a visualisation of loved ones, rather than himself, created some distance from Gordon's fears for a moment, providing a new platform from which to consider his options. Gordon described the little church in some detail as one of his daughters had got married there some years before. He went on to say how he would be able to see family and old friends that he hadn't seen for a long time, as well as how much he wanted to see his niece in her wedding dress.

Gordon was used to numerical scales as he used them with his medical team to rate his pain and activity levels. Therefore, we used a numerical scale of zero to 10 to rate how ready Gordon felt to go to the wedding, zero being not ready at all and 10 being totally ready. After the visualisation, Gordon was asked where he was on the scale and he said one out of 10. He was asked: 'Why a one and not a zero?' Gordon replied that he really wanted to go. Gordon was asked what it would take for him to get to a two out of 10, to which he replied he would need to know that his bag would not come loose. The aforementioned incident, where Gordon's bag had come loose, had affected him greatly, although it had only happened once. Consequently, via a series of questions about times when Gordon has been away from home and the bag had been safe, we built up a new story through which the time it came loose was the exceptionally unusual event, rather than something Gordon needed to worry about constantly.

We agreed that Gordon and his wife would go for another psychoeducation meeting at the nurse-led stoma clinic, partly for reassurance but also so Gordon could be sure to prepare as fully as possible before leaving for the wedding. Over the next two weeks, we worked through the scale to see how Gordon could get to the next step, and then the next. This took a very practical approach that included him talking to his family about his health difficulties, so he was reassured they would know the limits of what he could do. He also arranged two early exit points with family who lived close by, just in case he needed to leave early. After only three SFBT sessions, Gordon had reached seven out of 10 in terms of how ready he felt to go to the wedding. At the start of our next session, Gordon cheerfully explained that he had been to the wedding and had stayed well into the evening, recounting how beautiful and happy his niece looked and that he had enjoyed catching up with old friends and members of his family. It was reflected to Gordon that he seemed more confident and he said that he felt proud of himself and had been surprised how much everyone appreciated his efforts. He said he would try to attend more family gatherings and we agreed no further therapy was required at that time.

SFBT Four-week Group

Although SFBT is often delivered on a one-to-one basis, SFBT can also be delivered in a group setting, especially if group members have a common goal or some other shared experience. In a community mental health clinic, six people opted to join a new four-week SFBT course

(Continued)

to address their difficulties relating to a loss or bereavement. The group was designed to help the members learn new skills and adopt a future-orientated and optimistic outlook. As such, coping questions were asked throughout by the facilitator to encourage reflection and positive feedback was offered to model the approach to other members. The group structure was as follows:

Week One: Psychoeducation about SFBT approaches and setting expectations, including asking questions, such as 'What do you need to get from today to know coming to the group will be helpful?', followed by questions at the end, such as 'What will you take away from today?' and 'How has this been a different experience for you?'

Week Two: Goal setting, designing a personalised homework task and an individualised scale (some members used numbers or words, while others used metaphors such as the weather).

Week Three: Homework feedback, miracle question and scaling review. The homework feedback feature facilitated other members of the group to provide positive feedback to each member as they presented their progress, often offering their thoughts as to how each presenter had moved further up their scale. The group discussions, facilitated and guided by the practitioner, also led to some people revising their scales and adding more steps towards their goal as the route became clearer. This process relates to C. R. Snyder's Hope Theory (2000), which highlights that people need both pathways towards their goals and agency (self-belief) that the goal can be achieved. The group seemed to stimulate agency among themselves, which appeared to clarify the pathways members would need to take towards their goals. This process was further facilitated by the miracle question, before scales were reviewed a final time.

Week Four: Homework feedback and progress review. This final session included a review of key concepts and the progress members had made. The members also developed an action plan for themselves as to how they could continue their progress.

CONCLUSION

SFBT is a short-term, future-orientated, collaborative approach that aims to nurture agency and hopefulness through the skilled asking of particular questions, which are designed to instigate particular processes for the client. SFBT draws on a number of key techniques, such as scaling and questioning, to elicit new possibilities for the client to help them achieve specific goals.

DISCUSSION QUESTIONS

1. What personal characteristics of the therapist could help or hinder the delivery of SFBT?
2. Why is the collaborative element of SFBT so important?
3. Given the short-term and future orientation of SFBT, for whom might the approach not be suitable?
4. How could SFBT techniques be used within other approaches?

―――――――――――――― FURTHER READING ――――――――――――――

- de Shazer, S., Dolan, Y., Korman, H., Trepper, T., McCollum, E. E., & Berg, I. K. (2007). *More than miracles: The state of the art of solution-focused brief therapy.* London: The Haworth Press. ISBN: 9780789033987. An inviting and curiosity-satisfying book explaining the specialised use of language in SFBT.
- Kim, J. (2013). *Solution-focused brief therapy: A multicultural approach.* Thousand Oaks, CA: Sage. ISBN: 9781452256672. A practical overview of the essentials of SFBT from a multicultural perspective.
- Quick, E. K. (2013). *Solution focused anxiety management: A treatment and training manual.* Amsterdam: Academic Press. ISBN: 9780123944214. A clinician's guide to using SFBT approaches for anxiety, with flavours of CBT and ACT.
- Trepper, T. S., McCollum, E. E., De Jong, P., Korman, H., Gingerich, W., & Franklin, C. (2014). *Solution-focused therapy treatment manual for working with individuals.* Research Committee of the Solution Focused Brief Therapy Association. Available at: file://staffhome/staff_home0/55119606/Documents/RESEARCH/BI%20Book/Solution_Focused_Therapy_Treatment_Manual_for_Work.pdf
- Psychology Tools: Solution-Focused Therapy, Solution-Focused Brief Therapy and Brief Therapy Resources. Available at: https://psychologytools.com/solution-focused.html
- For more ideas, see The Centre for Solution Focused Practice at www.brief.org.uk/resources/brief-practice-notes/reading-guide

REFERENCES

Berg, I. K., & Dolan, Y. (2001). *Tales of solutions: A collection of hope-inspiring stories.* New York: W.W. Norton.

Berg, I. K., & Szabó, P. (2005). *Brief coaching for lasting solutions.* New York: W.W. Norton.

Davis, T. E., & Osborn, C. J. (2013). *Solution-focused school counselor: Shaping professional practice.* Abingdon, UK: Routledge.

de Shazer, S. (1978). Brief hypnotherapy of two sexual dysfunctions: The crystal ball technique. *American Journal of Clinical Hypnosis, 20*(3), 203–208.

de Shazer, S. (1985). *Keys to solutions in brief therapy.* New York: W.W. Norton.

de Shazer, S. (1988). *Clues: Investigating solutions in brief therapy.* New York: W.W. Norton.

de Shazer, S., Dolan, Y., Korman, H., Trepper, T., McCollum, E. E., & Berg, I. K. (2007). *More than miracles: The state of the art of solution-focused brief therapy.* London: The Haworth Press.

Franklin, C., Zhang, A., Froerer, A., & Johnson, S. (2017). Solution focused brief therapy: A systematic review and meta-summary of process research. *Journal of Marital and Family Therapy, 43*(1), 16–30.

Gingerich, W. J., & Peterson, L. T. (2013). Effectiveness of solution-focused brief therapy: A systematic qualitative review of controlled outcome studies. *Research on Social Work Practice, 23*(3), 266–283.

Gurman, A. (1981). Integrative marital therapy: Toward the development of an interpersonal approach. In S. Budman (Ed.), *Forms of brief therapy.* New York: Guilford Press.

Kim, J. S. (2008). Examining the effectiveness of solution-focused brief therapy: A meta-analysis. *Research on Social Work Practice, 18*(2), 107–116.

Kim, J. S., & Franklin, C. (2009). Solution-focused brief therapy in schools: A review of the outcome literature. *Children and Youth Services Review, 31*(4), 464–470.

Latham, G., & Locke, E. A. (2002). Building a practically useful theory of goal setting and task motivation. *American Psychologist, 57*, 705–717.

Maljanen, T., Härkänen, T., Virtala, E., Lindfors, O., Tillman, P., & Knekt, P. (2014). The cost-effectiveness of short-term psychodynamic psychotherapy and solution-focused therapy in the treatment of depressive and anxiety disorders during a three-year follow-up. *Open Journal of Psychiatry, 4*(3), 238.

National Institute for Health and Clinical Excellence (2004). *Improving supportive and palliative care for adults with cancer: The manual.* Guidance on Cancer Services. London: NICE.

National Institute for Health and Clinical Excellence (2009a). *Depression in adults: Recognition and management.* Nice Guideline (CG90). London: NICE.

National Institute for Health and Clinical Excellence (2009b). *Depression in adults with a chronic physical health problem.* Nice Guideline (CG91). London: NICE.

Sharry, J. (2007). *Solution-focused groupwork.* London: Sage.

Smock, S. A., Trepper, T. S., Wetchler, J. L., McCollum, E. E., Ray, R., & Pierce, K. (2008). Solution-focused group therapy for level 1 substance abusers. *Journal of Marital and Family Therapy, 34*(1), 107–120.

Snyder, C.R. (2000). *Handbook of hope: Theory, measures, and applications.* San Diego,CA: Academic Press.

Weiner-Davis, M., de Shazer, S., & Gingerich, W. J. (1987). Building on pre-treatment change to construct the therapeutic solution: An exploratory study. *Journal of Marital and Family Therapy, 13*(4), 359–363.

Zhang, A., Franklin, C., Currin-McCulloch, J., Park, S., & Kim, J. (2018). The effectiveness of strength-based, solution-focused brief therapy in medical settings: A systematic review and meta-analysis of randomized controlled trials. *Journal of Behavioral Medicine, 41*(2), 139–151.

5

SHORT-TERM FAMILY THERAPY

PANORAIA ANDRIOPOULOU

The main goal of therapy is to get people to behave differently and so to have different subjective experiences. (Haley, 1987, p. 56)

INTRODUCTION

Within individual therapeutic approaches, the assessment of intrapersonal processes that compromise a person's wellbeing will inform individualised case conceptualisations and lead to the development of therapeutic protocols. However, this chapter focuses on Systemic Models of Therapy, shifting the focus from the intrapsychic to the interpersonal, where the person's wellbeing is considered within the context of systemic interpersonal interactions. It is therefore essential to start with a definition of fundamental systemic concepts from the systemic school of thought before moving on to describe strategic approaches. It should be noted that there are different models of family therapy under the strategic umbrella, including the Mental Research Institute (MRI) or Palo Alto Model (Watzlawick, Weakland, & Fisch, 1974/2011), Haley and Madanes' Strategic Model (Haley, 1987), the Milan School of Family Therapy (Selvini Palazzoli, Cecchin, Prata, & Boscolo, 1978) and Szapocznik and colleagues' Brief Strategic Family Therapy (Szapocznik, Kurtines, Santisteban, & Rio, 1990). This chapter will focus on the MRI model of Strategic Family Therapy considering that the main theoretical ideas, which form the basis of all the strategic models, originate from the work of the Palo Alto or MRI group.

This chapter will discuss:

- Some core concepts of systemic therapy
- The MRI or Palo Alto Model of Brief Strategic Family Therapy
- The role of the MRI therapist
- The course of MRI therapy and its interventions
- The evaluation of the MRI model

This chapter aims to:

- familiarise the reader with some fundamental concepts of Systemic Family Therapy
- provide a coherent and straightforward narrative of the theoretical framework of the MRI model
- provide a clear, step-by-step account of how the model operates in practice

CORE CONCEPTS IN SYSTEMIC THERAPY

GENERAL SYSTEMS THEORY

The theoretical foundations of Systemic Family Therapy come from the General Systems Theory (GST), as developed by the biologist Ludwig von Bertalanffy in 1936 (Von Bertalanffy, 1950). Von Bertalanffy was interdisciplinary orientated and he believed that the same principles and laws govern all living systems, irrespective of their nature. He postulated that the whole is greater than the sum of its parts and that in order to understand how a system functions we need to study the relationships and the interactions between the parts. Following this line of reasoning, a family is more than the sum of the personalities and the intrapsychic worlds of its members. It also involves their relational and transactional patterns. Each system consists of subsystems (in the case of a family, these are the subsystem of the parental couple, the subsystem of siblings, etc.), which in turn consist of individual parts (e.g. family members). Each individual part of the system influences all other parts and subsystems as well as the system as a whole. Most crucially, even minor changes in any one part of the system will affect all the other parts. Consider, for example, the father of a family who has just started a new job and works mostly from home. He will probably need more time and space at the beginning to adjust to the new job. Therefore, his wife might undertake more responsibilities in the house or with the kids to give him this space and the kids might choose quieter activities in the afternoons.

According to von Bertalanffy, systems can be *closed* or *open*. Closed systems do not communicate with the surrounding environments and their boundaries are impermeable. Closed systems obey the laws of thermodynamics; they have a tendency to reach the simplest form, an equilibrium where no energy is produced by them. All living organisms, including families, are open systems. Open systems have semi-permeable boundaries which allow the influx and outflux of information from the surrounding environment. Open systems use these feedback loops to self-regulate and organise in order to avoid chaos and reach an *equilibrium* or *homeostasis*. As is the case for all open systems, families continually change, adapt and adjust as a result of new incoming information or new challenges, with an aim to reach homeostasis. To ensure homeostasis, certain rules are adopted and followed by family members. These rules (*homeostatic mechanisms*), provide a sense of order, coherence and organisation for the family and are essential in order for the family to function smoothly. Imagine, for example, a family consisting of the two parents and an 11-year-old daughter. The rule within this family is that the household chores are a female responsibility. The family members have embraced, and are happy with, this rule; the mother is the one who does all the housework whereas the father is the breadwin-ner, and the family functions in a patterned, predictable way. However, there are times when a family member breaks a rule or a change occurs and the rest of the system adapts to preserve homeostasis and the homeostatic mechanisms, sometimes at the expense of the family's wellbeing. Problems therefore arise when families fail to renegotiate the rules or when the attempted solutions to problems are unsuccessful. To return to the previous example, there might be a time when the mother of the family becomes seriously ill and needs to rest for a long period or takes a new job and needs to work away during the week. In keeping with the family rule, stating that household chores are a female responsibil-ity, the 11-year-old daughter is then left to do the cooking and to clean the house. This of course maintains homeostasis and might work in the short term, but the end result is that the daughter gets poorer grades at school, the father complains about the quality of the food and the mother admonishes the father for their daughter's school failure. As is evident from this example, very often families will resist or minimise change and will strive to maintain homeostasis, with detrimental consequences for the family. In systemic thinking, the difficulties of a family member – emotional distress, for example – develop as a means of restoring homeostasis and serve specific functions. In contrast, when families change, grow and adapt as a result of new information, they move towards *morphogenesis* (see Steinglass, 1987, for a detailed account of homeostatic and morphogenetic processes).

CYBERNETICS

This is a term coined by Norbert Wiener in 1948 that emerged as a result of a series of interdisciplinary conferences which took place in New York in the early 1940s with an aim to develop guidance systems for missiles and rockets through *feedback* mechanisms (Dallos & Draper, 2005). The idea was to create feedback loops through which systems would self-regulate by using new information. In this *first-order cybernetics*, it was assumed that the system was not influenced by the observer since the observer and the observed are separate from each other. In the practice of family therapy, this idea would imply that the therapist does not impact on or alter the family system in any way. It is rather assumed that the therapist can objectively observe the family and suggest changes while remaining outside the system itself. Subsequent, postmodern systemic theories moved away from that idea, postulating that it is impossible to observe the family system from the outside without becoming a participant of the system. In this *second-order cybernetics*, the therapist becomes part of the system, effecting change from the inside.

One of the major contributions of the GST and cybernetics is the idea of *circular causality*. Until then, the dominant idea was that most problems or symptoms are caused in a linear, stimulus–response fashion. Early psychoanalysts would mostly blame the mother for the 'symptoms' developed in the child, hence the development of outdated and stigmatising terms such as the 'schizophrenogenic mother' (see Neill, 1990, for a critical review). Circular causality removes the blame from the mother or any member of the family and offers a non-blaming, non-pathologising view of the problem. Consider the circular causation in the following example. A husband finds it very hard to express warm, affectionate feelings towards his wife, she then complains in an aggressive way about being emotionally deprived, which creates further barriers for the husband to express affectionate feelings. In this example who is to blame? Is it the husband or the wife? For the systemic therapist, none of the two is to blame. It is the repetitive interactional patterns that are the target of the intervention.

THE STRATEGIC APPROACH TO FAMILY THERAPY: THE MRI OR THE PALO ALTO MODEL

The Strategic Approach was developed in the 1950s at the Mental Research Institute (MRI) at Palo Alto, California. The model was mainly built upon the ideas of Bateson, Watzlawick and their colleagues. Bateson was studying families of individuals who had been diagnosed with schizophrenia and employed the cybernetics and systems theory to analyse the interactions and communication patterns of the family members. Watzlawick adopted some of Bateson's ideas and, along with his colleagues, he developed his communication theory, widely known as the Interactional View of Human behaviour. In 1967, Watzlawick, Beavin-Bavelas and Jackson published their influential book *The Pragmatics of Human Communication*, where they describe the rules and axioms that govern verbal and non-verbal family interactional patterns. Watzlawick and the MRI therapists adopted a constructivist perspective, according to which there is 'no fixed truth' when it comes to describing the reality but many different 'views' of reality. This approach is a non-blaming and non-pathologising approach.

Upon that reasoning, families have nothing inherently wrong with them and the only reason problems persist is mainly because they are maintained by current behavioural and interactional patterns. Therefore, the MRI therapist cannot 'educate' the family on more functional ways of communication like a cognitive behavioural therapist would do, since according to the constructivist view there is 'no one' ideal solution to the problem. Instead, the therapist intervenes to interrupt dysfunctional patterns of communication, respects the family's view of reality and 'trusts' the system in its ability to transform and move towards morphogenesis. The therapist intervenes to bring about change in the family's communication patterns without being able to predict the direction of this change.

The Strategic Approach focuses mainly on *solutions*; it is disinterested in the origin or the meaning of the symptom. The MRI therapists are not interested in determining *how* or *why* a problem has emerged; rather, they are interested in *what* is currently observable in the interactional patterns of the family (Wilder, 1979). They are also interested in examining how effective the problem-solving strategies and the communication patterns are when the family is dealing with crises. For the most part, families tend to use strategies that have been proven successful in the past. Problems arise when these strategies do not work anymore (or do not work when applied in the new situation) and instead of experimenting with novel solutions, the family is caught up in repetitive, negative feedback loops. As mentioned in the previous section, all families achieve homeostasis by adopting specific rules and patterns of communication. When a difficulty emerges, the family employs those rules to 'fix' the problem. The system changes only superficially at a behavioural level, not allowing for any restructuring or reorganisation. This is considered a *'first-order' change*.

On many occasions, the solution happens to be successful and no further problems arise. However, in other instances, this solution is not successful and the family needs to change their strategies, rules and patterns of communicating to deal with the new situation (*'second-order change'*). Problems occur when, instead of attempting a second-order change, the family applies 'more of the same' unsuccessful solutions. In other words, even though the attempted solutions do not work, the family continues to apply those solutions to solve the existing problem. The aim of the strategic interventions is to generate second-order change by interrupting dysfunctional interactional patterns and creating new interactions.

The defining characteristics of the model are as follows (Weakland, Fisch, Watzlawick, & Bodin, 1974):

1. *The model is problem/symptom-orientated*: Families come to therapy with a specific problem or complaint. The therapist's role is to work with the family to alleviate the presenting problem.
2. *The model adopts a non-pathologising and non-normative stance*: Symptoms are the result of the mishandling of everyday problems that arise in ordinary family life or of normal transitions in the family life cycle (e.g. marriage, birth of a child, retirement). It is the family's unsuccessful attempts to solve the problem that actually exacerbate and perpetuate it.
3. *The model assumes that attempted solutions perpetuate the problem*: The problem is maintained and often deteriorates as a result of the solutions that arise as a response to it, creating a positive feedback loop. The aim of therapy is to interrupt these dysfunctional feedback loops.
4. *The model is brief and goal-directed*: The therapist and the family work together to reach predetermined goals. According to MRI therapists, change is easier if the goals are small and clearly stated because small but definite changes very often lead to further, self-induced changes. The family is often allocated 'homework' assignments to make optimal use of time and promote positive change in real life. Therapy involves a maximum of 10 sessions.

5. *The model is fundamentally pragmatic*: The therapist's conceptualisations and interventions are based on the mere observation of interactions among the family members instead of on 'insight'. The therapist attempts to answer questions such as 'what' is going on in the system and 'how' the system continues to function like that, and has no interest as to 'why' the family system has reached this point.

6. *The model benefits from the use of an observation team*: This is a team of therapists who sit behind a one-way mirror in order to observe the family interactions and dynamics. The members of the team discuss their ideas and observations and share their reflections with the therapist and the family (see Andersen, 1987, for more information on the role of the reflecting teams).

Research on the effectiveness of the MRI model in its original form is rather limited. Nevertheless, there is ample indirect evidence either from research on systemic models that have incorporated strategic techniques, such as Szapocznik and colleagues' Brief Strategic Family model, which focuses on adolescents with drug use and related behavioural problems (e.g. Robbins, Feaster, Horigian, Puccinelli, Henderson, & Szapocznik, 2011; Robbins, Feaster, Horigian, Rohrbaugh et al., 2011), or from research on specific strategic interventions such as paradoxical interventions (e.g. Shoham-Salomon & Rosenthal, 1987) (see Sprenkle, 2012, for a more detailed review of outcome studies). The National Institute for Health and Care Excellence (NICE) recommends systemic approaches for a number of mental health problems, especially for children and young people (see, for example, Clinical Guidelines 28, 155, & 115 for depression, psychosis and harmful alcohol use, respectively – NICE, 2005, 2013, 2014).

THE THERAPIST'S STANCE

MRI therapists are very active and strategic in the sense that they are symptom- and goal-orientated. Families come to treatment experiencing specific problems and having specific complaints. Hence, the role of the MRI therapist is to take deliberate action to free the family from these problems as quickly and effectively as possible without exploring any deeper roots of difficulties or attempting to offer any insight. Promoting insight would presuppose that there is an absolute truth, which comes in direct opposition to MRI therapists' social constructionist philosophy. Instead, the therapeutic relationship is of a collaborative nature, with the therapist assuming a non-pathologising, not-knowing stance (Weakland et al., 1974). MRI therapists respect the family system and trust the system in its ability to reorganise itself and bring about change (Watzlawick et al., 1974/2011).

COURSE OF THERAPY

The MRI model follows a six-stage treatment protocol with some overlap among the stages (Weakland et al., 1974). The stages of treatment are outlined and considered below:

1. Introduction to treatment set-up
2. Assessment and clear definition of the problem(s)
3. Identification of the behaviour maintaining the problem ('attempted solutions')
4. Setting the goals of treatment
5. Selecting and making behavioural interventions
6. Termination of therapy

1. INTRODUCTION TO TREATMENT SET-UP

In the first session, the therapist's task is to introduce the family to the treatment set-up and obtain basic information about the family. The therapist informs the family of the length of the therapy (a maximum of 10 sessions). The therapist introduces the members of the observation team and explains their role and the benefits of their involvement. In many cases, the family is asked for permission to record sessions as they give the therapist and the team the opportunity to review past sessions and design future ones. Weber, McKeever and McDaniel (1985) have produced a step-by-step guide for the first family interview that is particularly practical, especially for inexperienced therapists.

2. ASSESSMENT AND CLEAR DEFINITION OF THE PROBLEM(S)

The therapist asks each individual family member to describe the problem in an attempt to assess how each member defines and experiences the problem. The therapist strives for clarity and specificity. Therefore, assessment questions could also include the following:

- 'How serious is the problem and how much does it affect the everyday functioning of the family?'
- 'When is the problem worse?'
- 'Are there any situations when the problem disappears or seems to be less serious?'
- 'Does the problem manifest itself in the presence of specific people?'
- 'Does the problem get better in the presence/absence of specific people?'
- 'Have you made any attempts to solve your problem in the past?'
- 'Have you seen a therapist before?'
- 'Why have you decided to ask for help now?'
- 'What do you do now because of the problem that you would like to stop doing?'
- 'What have you stopped doing because of the problem?'
- 'How would things be different if the problem disappeared?'
- 'If it disappeared, how would you know it's not there?'

The miracle question from the solution-focused approach could also be used (see Chapter 4).

3. IDENTIFICATION OF ATTEMPTED SOLUTIONS

In this stage of therapy, the therapist asks questions to assess the attempted solutions. For example: How has the family tried to solve the problem? Have they tried one or more solutions and were there any solutions that alleviated the problem even if only temporarily?

According to Fisch, Weakland and Segal (1982, p. 128), there are five common types of attempted solutions:

1. People frequently attempt to force something that can only occur spontaneously (e.g. they try to fix or control a bodily function, such as sleep or sexual performance, failing to accept that fluctuations are normal).
2. People frequently attempt to master a fearful event by postponing it (e.g. they frequently avoid fearful situations and, as a result, they create and maintain cognitions of vulnerability).
3. People frequently attempt to reach accord through opposition (e.g. a parent expects their adolescent son to comply by overstating their power or a spouse attempts to receive affection by protesting rather than requesting).
4. People frequently attempt to obtain compliance through volunteerism (e.g. a father expects his son not only to comply with the rules he has chosen, but also to be happy about it and to want to comply; or a wife expects her husband not only to guess what her needs are without telling him, but also to meet these needs in a satisfactory way).
5. People frequently attempt to decrease an accuser's suspicions by attempting to defend themselves (e.g. a couple is caught in a game of accuser/defender, where the husband accuses the wife of having an affair and she tries to defend herself only to confirm her husband's suspicions).

TOP TIP

Always request specificity and clarity when you assess the presenting problem(s) and the attempted solution(s). Specificity is also key when determining therapeutic goals.

---

4. SETTING THE GOALS OF TREATMENT

Given the brief nature of strategic family therapy, goals should be stated in an explicit way. The goals should be described in behavioural terms in order to be both observable and measurable. Sometimes couples or families present to therapy with an undefined goal. Consider the following goal: 'We would like to improve our communication'. What does the family mean by an improved communication? Is what they mean the same as what the therapist has in mind? How would the therapist know if their communication is improving in the course of therapy? It is therefore really important to explicitly define goals and transform them into behaviours by asking the clients: 'How would you know that your communication has improved?', 'What would you *do* differently?', 'How would your everyday life change as a result of your better communication?'

The clients' answers to these questions will provide the therapist with a list of concrete goals. It is of course equally important that the goals are attainable in the course of treatment and are relevant to the problem(s) identified in the assessment phase. For MRI therapists, even small behavioural changes can be very important as they can work in a domino-like fashion. The idea is that one change will potentially lead to a number of other, self-induced behavioural shifts that will ultimately result in second-order change.

5. INTERVENTIONS

MRI therapists, influenced by the hypnotic work of Milton Erickson (see Erickson & Keeney, 2006), employ implicit or indirect interventions with an aim to interrupt repetitive, dysfunctional interactions and generate change.

REFRAMING

In their chapter 'The Gentle Art of Reframing', Watzlawick and colleagues (1974/2011) define reframing as an intervention in which the therapist helps the client attach an alternative meaning/frame to a situation – a new frame that fits the data equally well, changing entirely both the interpretation of the situation and the emotional experience of the client. So, even though the situation does not really change, or may even be unchangeable, the way the person experiences the situation does change and once the client manages to perceive the situation through an alternative frame, it is really hard to go back to the former way of thinking. Milan therapists (see Boscolo, Cecchin, Hoffman, & Penn, 1987) developed this technique further by attaching a positive meaning (*positive connotation*) to a behaviour or symptom. Clients do not necessarily need to adopt the new frame exactly, nor does the new frame need to reflect the actual truth.

The aim of reframing is to bring into the family system new information that will initiate systemic change – a first-order change if it is at a behavioural level or a second-order change if it is at a family rule level. In any case, the family will make its own meaning and will use this new information in its own way. Therefore, the direction of the change is not always predictable. Consider the following case example. A couple comes to therapy because one party complains that his partner has changed since they first met. He reports that his partner used to be carefree and very talkative and now is always preoccupied and overly concerned with how to keep the house tidy, which is interpreted as being indifferent and aloof. The therapist could reframe the behaviour, suggesting that the preoccupation with the cleanliness of the house is driven by a desire to provide a warm, welcoming environment in which they can relax when returning from a difficult day at work. Milan therapists also employ *circular questioning* to unveil the interactive patterns of the family system, thus allowing the system to reframe the problem itself without the therapist providing a reframe. The interested reader can refer to the seminal paper by Selvini Palazzoli, Boscolo, Cecchin and Prata (1980) on hypothesising–circularity–neutrality.

TOP TIP

It is essential to assess your client's worldviews. Your interventions will be more well received and more successful if you take into consideration your client's conceptual framework and language.

PARADOXICAL INTERVENTIONS

Paradoxical interventions involve instructing the family members to adopt behaviours that appear to come in direct opposition to the goals of treatment. Paradoxical inter-ventions can be very powerful techniques, bringing about quick and extraordinary change.

SYMPTOM/BEHAVIOUR PRESCRIPTION OR WORSENING OF A SYMPTOM

For example, the parents of an adolescent who is behaving in an adult-like manner, push-ing for more liberties, might be given the instruction to encourage the adolescent to behave in even more adult-like ways, assuming all the responsibilities of an adult role (e.g. paying bills, cooking, cleaning the house). The parents, on the other hand, assume a child-like role, asserting no control over the adolescent and contributing nothing to the household. In this way, the symptom or the behaviour places the person (the adolescent in this case) at a disadvantage. His behaviour costs him more than it earns. Similarly, a couple who complain about everyday arguments might be given the instruction to have more intense arguments, more often and of longer duration. In an attempt to argue more, the couple become so tired of arguing that they abandon arguing altogether. Alternatively, they might discover that arguing 'on prescription' is not 'fun' anymore. In any case, the therapist offers the client a 'therapeutic double bind' where progress is achieved no matter how the client responds.

RESTRAINING TECHNIQUE OR 'GOING SLOW'

The therapist stresses to the family the importance of 'going slow' or expressing their con-cern for 'things moving too fast'. This technique is particularly useful for families whose attempted solution is 'trying too hard'. It is usually employed in the first few sessions with an aim to reduce the family's sense of urgency. By doing so, the family relaxes their attempts to solve the problem, breaking the vicious cycles of interactions (Fisch et al., 1982). A family member who experiences depression, for example, might be instructed to slow down their improvement because 'things are moving too fast'. The rest of the family might then give up unhelpful behaviours, such as continuously noticing and discussing depressive symptoms and suggesting solutions.

DISADVANTAGES OF IMPROVEMENT

Another way to interrupt attempted solutions and reduce the sense of urgency is by getting the family to list the disadvantages or dangers of improvement. In many cases, the family realise that the improvement will not be as pleasant as they might have believed and may abandon their attempted solutions.

In some cases, the family might even be informed by the therapist that their problem is so serious and deep-rooted that no therapist could possibly be of any assistance. This is a particularly powerful technique with families who ask for immediate help but at the same time claim that nothing has worked for them in the past, such as families with a member who has had multiple hospitalisations or families with chronic substance abuse issues. This kind of instruction will very often lead the family to disobey the therapist or prove that the therapist is wrong, thus changing the pattern of interaction or abandoning the undesirable behaviour altogether (Watzlawick et al., 1974/2011). In any case, these interventions provide families with a sense of control by changing the direction or the intensity of the problem.

TOP TIP

Aim for small changes. Changing the pattern of interactions even slightly will 'shake' the family system and will initiate further changes and develop virtuous cycles.

---

6. TERMINATION OF THERAPY

The course of therapy and potential improvements are reviewed. The therapist reminds the family that the therapy is only a starting point on which they can build. In contrast, when the family is negativistic, the therapist appears to be pessimistic about the future. In both cases, the therapist's aim is to extend their therapeutic influence beyond the 10 sessions. Families are usually contacted by telephone three months after the termination of therapy for a follow-up interview (Weakland et al., 1974).

EVALUATION OF THE MODEL

As mentioned earlier, the model is based on non-pathologising and collaborative principles, which makes it suitable for families from diverse cultural backgrounds, especially as MRI therapists make no rigid assumptions about how a 'normal' family should function. Another strength of the model is the fact that the family and the therapist(s) work together in a collaborative fashion towards clear and agreed therapeutic goals, which for the most part are set by the family. The model also benefits from the presence of the reflective team, which allows for more objective observations of the family dynamics.

At the same time, the model's critics consider paradoxical interventions manipulative, or even deceptive, as the rationale for their use is not explained to the family. However, MRI therapists believe that influence is an inherent element of all human communication. Clients notably seek help for specific problems or aspects of their lives that they are dissatisfied with, assigning the therapist with the task to influence their thoughts, feelings and behaviours towards agreed and desirable goals (Weakland et al., 1974).

──────────── STORY FROM PRACTICE ────────────

The Brown family

Background information

The Brown family consists of the parents and two adult sons, aged 18 and 22. Mr Brown is a computer specialist and Mrs Brown is a librarian. Both of the sons are studying at university, at undergraduate and postgraduate levels, respectively. The older son is also working part-time as a research assistant. The family reports that problems started when the paternal grandfather, who managed the family's financial issues and made most of the decisions, passed away. Mr B assumed all the financial responsibility, adopting Scrooge-like behaviour. At the same time, Mrs B started working, even though this is something she did not really want to do. The younger son suffers from asthma attacks and he does not respond to medication well. The family decided to ask for the help of a family therapist when the doctor suggested that the asthma attacks could be of a psychosomatic nature.

Presenting problems

Mr B feels that his family does not respect him anymore and that they ignore his wishes and his feelings. He thinks that his wife spends a lot of money and that the family could easily go bankrupt if they did not plan carefully (even though the family is not experiencing financial difficulties and could be considered wealthy). He complains that his wife and children avoid him.

Mrs B and the sons complain about the fact that the father has been transformed from a happy, relaxed and open-handed person to a stingy, authoritarian father. Mrs B believes that things became worse since she started working; the son's asthma attacks became more severe and more frequent and she has bigger and more heated arguments with her husband.

Attempted solutions

Mr B tries to get the family to respect and obey him by exerting a very tight financial control. As a result, the younger son will never go out with his friends because he does not have any financial autonomy. He spends most of his time at home. Mrs B and the older son have been obliged to contribute most of their salaries to cover household expenses.

Both Mrs B and her sons ignore Mr B's requests. They never 'obey' him, as he says. Instead, when his requests seem unreasonable to them they respond with ironic comments. They will go to great lengths to avoid an open confrontation with him. Therefore, when the father is in the sitting room, the three of them will stay in the kitchen. The family has even stopped having meals together.

A conceptualisation based on the MRI model could be the following: After the death of his father, Mr B starts feeling the pressure of assuming financial responsibility and of making important decisions for his family. Feeling insecure under the pressure of his new role, he behaves in a domineering way. The more controlling Mr B becomes the more the members of his family rebel, and the more they rebel (by being distant or sarcastic) the more controlling he becomes, establishing a vicious cycle.

PRACTITIONER TAKE HOME MESSAGES

- Respect the family's perspective and trust its potential for transformation.
- Always remember that there is no linear causation for the formation of problems. None of the family members is to blame for dysfunctional interactions.
- Problems are oftentimes perpetuated by the family's attempts to solve them.
- Abandoning these habitual solutions or experimenting with new ones can lead to problem resolution.

CONCLUSION

The contribution of the MRI therapists is unquestionable as not only did they offer a comprehensive account of the axioms of human communication, but they also formulated a theory of problem formation and resolution. As many of the techniques of the model have been found to be effective, either in isolation or when integrated with other systemic models, and given its brief and potentially cost-effective nature, more systematic empirical research is essential.

DISCUSSION QUESTIONS

1. Critically consider the advantages and disadvantages of paradoxical interventions.
2. Consider how the methods and techniques of Strategic Family Therapy can be incorporated into other family therapy models (e.g. Cognitive Behavioural Family Therapy).
3. Based on the information provided for the Brown family, make a list of the potential treatment goals and devise a treatment plan incorporating relevant interventions.

FURTHER READING

- Dallos, R., & Draper, R. (2010). *An introduction to family therapy: Systemic theory and practice*. Maidenhead: McGraw-Hill Education (UK).
- Goldenberg, H., & Goldenberg, I. (2012). *Family therapy: An overview*. Boston, MA: Cengage Learning.
- Haley, J. (1987). *Problem-solving therapy*. San Francisco, CA: Jossey-Bass.

- Watzlawick, P., Weakland, J. H., & Fisch, R. (1974/2011). *Change: Principles of problem formation and problem resolution.* New York: W.W. Norton.
- Fisch, R., Weakland, J. H., & Segal, L. (1982). *The tactics of change: Doing therapy briefly.* San Francisco, CA: Jossey-Bass.
- Nardone, G., & Salvini, A. (2007). *The strategic dialogue: Rendering the diagnostic interview a real therapeutic intervention.* London: Karnac Books.
- Nardone, G., & Watzlawick, P. (1993). *The art of change: Strategic therapy and hypnotherapy without trance.* San Francisco, CA: Jossey-Bass.
- Mental Research Institute: https://mri.org
- Association for Family Therapy and Systemic Practice: www.aft.org.uk/view/index.html
- Institute of Family Therapy: www.ift.org.uk

REFERENCES

Andersen, T. (1987). The reflecting team: Dialogue and meta-dialogue in clinical work. *Family Process, 26*(4), 415–428.

Boscolo, L., Cecchin, G., Hoffman, L., & Penn, P. (1987). *Milan systemic family therapy: Conversations in theory and practice.* New York: Basic Books.

Dallos, R., & Draper, R. (2005). *An introduction to family therapy: Systemic theory and practice.* Milton Keynes: Open University Press.

Erickson, B. A., & Keeney, B. (Eds.). (2006). *Milton H. Erickson, M.D.: An American healer.* Sedona, AZ: Ringing Rocks Press.

Fisch, R., Weakland, J. H., & Segal, L. (1982). *The tactics of change.* San Francisco, CA: Jossey-Boss.

Haley, J. (1987). *Problem-solving therapy.* San Francisco, CA: Jossey-Bass.

National Institute for Health and Clinical Excellence (2005). *Depression in children and young people: Identification and management.* NICE Guideline (CG28). London: NICE.

National Institute for Health and Clinical Excellence (2013). *Psychosis and schizophrenia in children and young people: Recognition and management.* NICE Guideline (CG155). London: NICE.

National Institute for Health and Clinical Excellence (2014). *Alcohol-use disorders: Diagnosis, assessment and management of harmful drinking and alcohol dependence.* NICE Guideline (CG115). London: NICE.

Neill, J. (1990). Whatever became of the schizophrenogenic mother? *American Journal of Psychotherapy, 4*(4), 499–505.

Robbins, M. S., Feaster, D. J., Horigian, V. E., Puccinelli, M. J., Henderson, C., & Szapocznik, J. (2011). Therapist adherence in brief strategic family therapy for adolescent drug abusers. *Journal of Consulting and Clinical Psychology, 79*(1), 43.

Robbins, M. S., Feaster, D. J., Horigian, V. E., Rohrbaugh, M., Shoham, V., Bachrach, K., ... & Vandermark, N. (2011). Brief strategic family therapy versus treatment as usual: Results of a multisite randomized trial for substance using adolescents. *Journal of Consulting and Clinical Psychology, 79*(6), 713.

SHORT-TERM FAMILY THERAPY

Selvini Palazzoli M., Boscolo, L., Cecchin, G., & Prata, G. (1980). Hypothesizing—Circularity—Neutrality: Three guidelines for the conductor of the session. *Family Process, 19*(1), 3–12.

Selvini Palazzoli, M., Cecchin, G., Prata, G., & Boscolo, L. (1978). *Paradox and counterparadox: A new model in the therapy of the family in schizophrenic transaction*. New York: Jason Aronson.

Shoham-Salomon, V., & Rosenthal, R. (1987). Paradoxical interventions: A meta-analysis. *Journal of Consulting and Clinical Psychology, 55*(1), 22–28.

Sprenkle, D. H. (2012). Intervention research in couple and family therapy: A methodological and substantive review and an introduction to the special issue. *Journal of Marital and Family Therapy, 38*(1), 3–29.

Steinglass, P. (1987). A system's view of family interaction and psychopathology. In T. Jacob, (Ed.), *Family interaction and psychopathology* (pp. 25–65). New York: Springer US.

Szapocznik, J., Kurtines, W., Santisteban, D. A., & Rio, A. T. (1990). Interplay of advances between theory, research, and application in treatment interventions aimed at behavior problem children and adolescents. *Journal of Consulting and Clinical Psychology, 58*(6), 696–703.

Von Bertalanffy, L. (1950). The theory of open systems in physics and biology. *Science, 111*(2872), 23–29. doi:10.1126/science.111.2872.23

Watzlawick, P., Beavin-Bavelas, J., & Jackson, D. D. (1967). *The pragmatics of human communication*. London: Faber & Faber.

Watzlawick, P., Weakland, J. H., & Fisch, R. (1974/2011). *Change: Principles of problem formation and problem resolution*. New York: W.W. Norton.

Weakland, J. H., Fisch, R., Watzlawick, P., & Bodin, A. M. (1974). Brief therapy: Focused problem resolution. *Family Process, 13*(2), 141–168.

Weber, T., McKeever, J. E., & McDaniel, S. H. (1985). A beginner's guide to the problem-oriented first family interview. *Family Process, 24*(3), 357–364.

Wiener, N. (1948). Cybernetics. *Scientific American, 179*(5), 14–19.

Wilder, C. (1979). The Palo Alto group: Difficulties and directions of the interactional view for human communication research. *Human Communication, 5*(2), 171–186.

6

SHORT-TERM ACCEPTANCE AND COMMITMENT THERAPY

KATY ROE

INTRODUCTION

This chapter will discuss Acceptance and Commitment Therapy (ACT), which was developed by Hayes, Strosahl and Wilson (1999) to offer a new approach to psychological therapy, one that works on the assumption that the ordinary psychological processes of the human mind cause suffering – a term they call 'destructive normality'. In this chapter, we will explore how ACT can influence people in their day-to-day lives as well as:

- introduce the model and the six core processes that promote psychological flexibility
- explore an overview of the principles and philosophy of ACT
- consider the variety of ways in which ACT can be used with clients in therapeutic work and beyond the therapy room.

ACT has been described as:

An empirically-based psychological intervention that uses acceptance and mindfulness strategies with commitment and behaviour-change strategies to increase psychological flexibility. (Hayes, 2009)

In essence, this means that people can learn to develop a different relationship with their own internal experiences and live a life that is meaningful to them. *Psychological flexibility* describes the ability to persist or desist in behaviour when it enables us to live the life we want to live based upon what matters to us personally. The Hexaflex Model (see Figure 6.1) is unique to ACT and encompasses six core concepts that are believed to contribute to increasing psychological flexibility. This diagram can be a helpful aid when therapists are new to the model and provide a framework for understanding how all the skills interconnect.

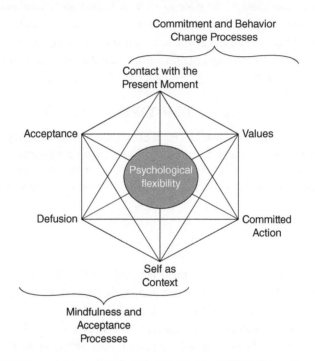

Figure 6.1 The six core components of the Hexaflex Model of ACT (© Steven C. Hayes, used with permission)

THEORETICAL INTRODUCTION

The development of ACT took place over two decades, with scientific work undertaken to ensure that the robust philosophy can be applied in theory and practice. A focus upon the context and function of behaviour (including private experiences) enables the approach to be transdiagnostic (i.e. it applies to more than one condition). Essentially, the role for the therapist is to help the client develop skills that will allow them to make space for previously unwanted internal experiences (what they may have labelled as symptoms) and to identify and practise their Values (what gives our lives meaning and purpose).

ACT, Dialectical Behaviour Therapy (DBT), Functional Analytic Psychotherapy (FAP), Mindfulness-Based Cognitive Therapy (MBCT) and Mindfulness-Based Stress Reduction (MBSR) are often described as third-wave cognitive behaviour therapy approaches. The first wave of behaviour therapy in the 1950s and 1960s was linked to classical (respondent) conditioning and operant conditioning principles, which involved behaviours that can be modified through the association of stimuli or by the effect they produce (i.e. reward or punishment). These approaches were criticised heavily for not acknowledging the important function of thoughts and belief systems with regards to influencing behaviour. The second wave emerged in the 1970s and included working with cognition as part of invoking behaviour change. The main focus of such work was challenging or disputing 'dysfunctional' and 'irrational' thinking patterns in favour of more positive and rational ones. In the late 1980s, Steven Hayes and colleagues developed the model we now understand as ACT, with a focus on the function, rather than the form, of thoughts.

TOP TIPS

To understand the theoretical underpinnings of ACT, you can read Russ Harris's outtake from The Happiness Trap (at http://thehappinesstrap.com/upimages/the_house_of_ACT.pdf), which provides a very readable introduction to the foundations of ACT, including Functional Contextualism, Applied Behavioural Analysis and Relational Frame Theory (RFT).

RFT is a psychological theory of human language. Within RFT it is understood that the building block of human language and higher cognition is 'relating', i.e. the human ability to create bidirectional links between things without these being explicitly taught (Hayes, Barnes-Holmes, & Roche, 2001; Harris & Aisbett, 2014).

By December 2016, 171 randomised controlled trials (RCTs) of ACT had been published. The American Psychological Association (APA), Society of Clinical Psychology (Division 12), identified that ACT shows 'strong' research support for the field of chronic pain and 'modest' research support for depression, mixed anxiety, psychosis and obsessive-compulsive disorder (see Forman et al., 2007; McCracken & Vowles, 2014). ACT has also been found to be helpful in a range of different settings outside the therapy room, including impacting on the spread of Ebola in Sierra Leone by helping whole communities to worship in a way that reduced the spread of infection (Rhodes, 2014), to a focus on workplace wellbeing and distilling down the principles of ACT into a three-session, manualised approach (Flaxman, Bond, & Livheim, 2013). The ACT model focuses on a much broader definition of psychological distress and wellbeing than commonly conceptualised by diagnostic labels.

The opening remark in the original ACT text states: 'the single most remarkable fact of human existence is how hard it is for human beings to be happy' (Hayes, Strosahl, &

Wilson, 1999, p. 1). In Western society, we have bought into the ideology that good mental health is synonymous with happiness and made assumptions that, by their nature, humans are and should be psychologically healthy. ACT offers an alternative assumption: that the psychological processes of a 'normal' human mind are often destructive and eventually can create problems for us all. Given the way in which humans have evolved, our minds have a natural tendency to a negative bias. It also defaults to psychological inflexibility as we enter into a struggle to escape from, alter or avoid our own thoughts, feelings, bodily sensations and memories (stuff that feels negative and/ or threatening) and in the process of doing so, lose sight of what matters in the bigger picture. The aim of ACT is to change our relationship with our difficult thoughts and feelings so that we no longer experience them as *'signs of threat or danger'* or *'symptoms of pathology'*, but rather as just transient internal experiences such as sensations in the body or images in the mind.

The philosophy behind ACT recognises that human suffering exists for everyone and attributes this in part to two specific processes that are unique to the human species:

1. *Experiential avoidance*: humans attempt to avoid, control or alter their own internal experiences (thoughts, feelings, memories and bodily sensation), unlike other animal species.
2. *Cognitive fusion*: this means we take language literally and, in doing so, language functions to create rigid verbal rules and information that we perceive as *'truths'*, for example, 'I am *unlovable*' becomes a fact rather than being seen as a form of evaluative thinking.

EVALUATION

The ACT approach is suitable for a range of human issues and multiple problems. ACT is delivered as an experiential approach to therapy, which means that within the sessions there are many exercises that clients can undertake to get a felt sense of a particular issue as opposed to a logical understanding. This is at the very heart of an ACT approach and offers a great amount of flexibility and creativity within the sessions. There are numerous exercises and metaphors that can be used in sessions, which are consistent with the pragmatic philosophy of the model, reflecting its roots in behaviour analysis. The focus on Values is broadly applicable to adults in a cross-cultural context.

ACT has been successfully delivered in various formats and clinical and non-clinical settings. For example, when working with adolescents in secondary schools, Hayes and Ciarocchi (2015) talk more of 'Vitality', along with Values, and the Discoverer, Noticer and Advisor parts of ourselves, as this is a developmental model of ACT. The use of *therapy* may be substituted for *training* when introduced in work-based settings (e.g. Flaxman, Bond, & Livheim, 2013). Alternatively, there are numerous protocols for ACT that aim to work with a diverse range of people experiencing clinical problems. Guy Meadows (2014) specialises in ACT for insomnia. He has devised a range of delivery options from one-day workshops to online training and the use of phone Apps. Professor Neil Frude has produced a four-session, community-based psychoeducation programme which is delivered across six of seven health boards in Wales in local village halls and supermarket cafés (Cartwright & Hooper, 2017). Strosahl, Robinson and Gustavsson's (2012) work in primary care employing Focused Acceptance and Commitment Therapy (FACT) has proven the success of brief behavioural interventions. Within the physical health field there are protocols for chronic pain (Vowles, Wetherell, & Sorrell, 2009) and diabetes self-management (Gregg, Callaghan, & Hayes, 2007), and in severe and enduring mental health difficulties, such as psychosis, four-session interventions have been developed (Bach & Hayes, 2002). This illustrates that the model is flexible enough to be used across the lifespan and within different clinical and non-clinical settings.

Some clients are looking for an outcome that is incompatible with an ACT approach (e.g. the removal of symptoms or an exclusive exploration of the past) and in those cases I am comfortable referring clients on to other therapeutic approaches, such as CAT or more generic cognitive behavioural therapy.

PRACTICAL GUIDE

I work as a clinical psychologist in private practice and see many clients who have tried other approaches, which they report have not been helpful in the longer term. ACT seems to appeal because clients have got to a point where they are tired of struggling and suffering. I often reframe the difficulties my clients bring to therapy as more an issue of 'stuckness' rather than the label they were given or have had ascribed to themselves (e.g. 'I'm too anxious' or 'I'm not confident enough' or 'I have XYZ disorder').

The initial assessment session would follow a typical therapeutic assessment process in terms of allowing the client the opportunity to tell the story that led them to seeking therapy. I use a variety of generic mental health or physical health outcome measures, some process measures specific to ACT and mindfulness skills. For example, the Valued Living Questionnaire (Wilson et al., 2010) and the Acceptance and Action Questionnaire (AAQ-II, Bond et al., 2011) or the Mindful Attention Awareness Scale (Brown & Ryan, 2003) can all be used to explore mechanisms of change within the model, rather than evaluate symptom reduction. ACT makes it clear that the therapist and client are in the same boat, which means that appropriate self-disclosure is a fundamental part of therapy.

There are a number of different ways to conceptualise clients' difficulties and what might be a helpful alternative approach. The Psychological Flexibility Matrix, developed by Kevin Polk (Polk & Schoendorff, 2014; see Figure 6.2), is a user-friendly way of introducing the three different aspects of ourselves and highlights the tension that exists between experiential avoidance and moving towards a life that will be more fulfilling.

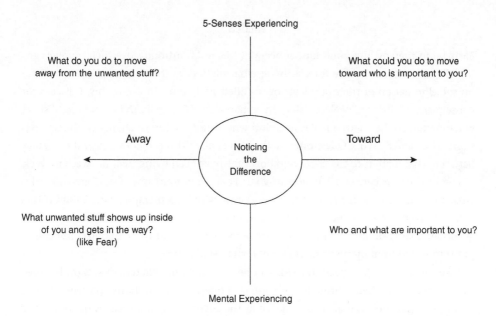

5-Senses Experiencing

What do you do to move
away from the unwanted stuff?

What could you do to move
toward who is important to you?

Away

Noticing
the
Difference

Toward

What unwanted stuff shows up inside
of you and gets in the way?
(like Fear)

Who and what are important to you?

Mental Experiencing

Figure 6.2   The Psychological Flexibility Matrix Diagram (© Kevin L. Polk, used with permission)

CREATIVE HOPELESSNESS

The start of therapeutic work, and an integral part of psychoeducation, involves under-mining the client's 'control' agenda. In ACT, the process of *creative hopelessness* is typically explored via three simple questions:

1. What have you tried to solve the problems you are experiencing?
2. How has that worked for you?
3. What has that cost you?

Numerous experiential exercises can be used to illustrate this point with clients. One of the most commonly cited is the 'Chinese Finger Traps'. Clients put their two index fingers in the tube-like structure and try to pull them out. It illustrates how they become trapped further by struggling and trying to pull away. We also use metaphors in session to illustrate the six core concepts and to address certain points effectively, without becoming ensnared in language and logic. 'The Quicksand' is an ideal metaphor to use early on in therapeutic work, as we ask clients to consider what they would do if they found them-selves in quicksand? They recognise that their initial reaction, understandably, would be to struggle and that this would cause them to sink in deeper and deeper as they try to escape, but the alternative, counterintuitive approach would be to get in full contact with the quicksand, spreading their surface area and preventing the sinking process.

VALUES

Early on in therapy, the important concept of 'Values' is introduced, which involves giving clients a clear rationale for clarifying what matters to them, as opposed to a focus on the elimination of their problems or so-called symptoms. In doing this, I discuss the consequences when we neglect Values in certain areas of life. Clarifying and establishing what matters to the client enables us to influence the direction of change in therapy sessions. The Valued Living Questionnaire (Wilson et al., 2010) provides a clear discrepancy between what matters to the client and how they have been living their life week to week.

The distinction between Values and goals is an important one. Goals are often discussed in generic CBT; however, the beauty of working as a therapist with Values is that it can be lived and embodied in that very moment. ACT uses the term *Values* to refer to 'a chosen quality of purposeful action that can never be obtained as an object but can be put into action from moment to moment' (Hayes et al., 1999).

Take the Value of 'connection'. This can be achieved immediately in session between the therapist and client through eye contact, honesty and emotional presence to one another. Connection can also be achieved as the client or therapist leaves the office and makes eye contact with the first person they meet and smile at. It might also be in the form of a phone call to a friend – just to say we were thinking of them. The value of connection and connectedness can be lived in a myriad of ways. However, it is not something that will ever be fully achieved but, like a direction on a compass, will always provide a position to return to.

In therapy, we are still interested in goals. As part of ACT home practice (homework), setting SMART (specific, measurable, achievable, realistic and time-framed) goals can be used to achieve Values-based action. For example, wanting to feel more connected to my children might lead me to plan to set aside an hour to play a board game with them rather than spending two evenings per week doing housework. In this way, the goal is tangible and can be directly related to the value that reinforces it. Goals are carried out as part of *committed action*, which is another core process in ACT, one that allows us to actually live and demonstrate our Values.

One way to help clients to get in touch with their Values is to provide them with a list of core values to establish 10 that are meaningful to them. Often this process may reveal key areas of emotional pain that are linked to the things they value and which they may be neglecting. See Figure 6.3 for an example of core values.

Above and Beyond	Dependability	Individuality	Reason
Acceptance	Depth	Industry	Recognition
Accessibility	Determination	Informal	Recreation
Accomplishment	Determined	Innovation	Refined
Accountability	Development	Innovative	Reflection

Accuracy	Devotion	Inquisitive	Relationships
Accurate	Devout	Insight	Relaxation
Achievement	Different	Insightful	Reliability
Activity	Differentiation	Insiration	Reliable
Adaptability	Dignity	Integrity	Resilience
Adventure	Diligence	Intelligence	Resolute
Adventurous	Direct	Intensity	Resolution
Affection	Directness	International	Reslove
Affective	Discipline	Intuition	Resourceful
Aggressive	Discovery	Intuitive	Resourcefulness
Agility	Discreation	Invention	Respect

Figure 6.3 An outtake example of a list of core values

MINDFULNESS

Mindfulness involves a number of skills, including: observing, describing, acting with awareness, focused attention, acceptance without judgement, non-reactivity to internal experiences and non-attachment (Sahdra, Ciarrochi, & Parker, 2016). Mindfulness within the ACT model involves paying attention to our here-and-now experiences, and by doing so facilitates our ability to move towards our Values. Figure 6.4 is a mini act formulation which explains the rationale for cultivating Mindfulness in our clients and how it directly impacts upon Values. There is also plenty of scientific evidence to support the physical and emotional benefits of Mindfulness for our wellbeing and we can share this evidence with our clients to encourage practice. Within ACT, we use Mindfulness as a means to support and clear a pathway towards Values that are more consistent with our behaviour and living.

COMMITTED ACTION

A committed-action aligns with the client's goals, which are connected to their values and are meaningful and possible to achieve, Committed-actions can lead to healthy actions that enrich their lives. Within a contextual framework, behaviours are not labelled or judged as 'right', 'wrong' or 'disordered'. It is the function of that behaviour we are interested in. The function is often an attempt to alter, escape or avoid aversive internal experiences. As such, a client who presents with excessive hand washing, which they have labelled as 'an OCD behaviour' or as 'not normal', will be encouraged to examine whether this behaviour is compatible or incompatible with the life they want to lead. The criterion of workability is extremely important in the ACT model as clients often get tied

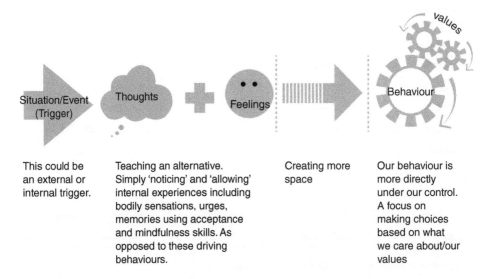

This could be an external or internal trigger.

Teaching an alternative. Simply 'noticing' and 'allowing' internal experiences including bodily sensations, urges, memories using acceptance and mindfulness skills. As opposed to these driving behaviours.

Creating more space

Our behaviour is more directly under our control. A focus on making choices based on what we care about/our values

Figure 6.4 Mini act formulation of thoughts, feelings and behaviour

up in the rights and wrongs. This allows them to explore the fact that, in some instances, such behaviour can be considered adaptive (e.g. if you were a brain surgeon). The use of committed action is a way of asking and teaching clients to carry out their Values on a day-to-day and week-to-week basis.

WILLINGNESS (AKA ACCEPTANCE)

Clients are introduced to the idea that the alternative or antidote to Experiential Avoidance is a stance of willingness towards their own internal experiences. They are encouraged to recognise that their thoughts, feelings, bodily sensations and memories are transient experiences and that they can be an observer to those experiences rather than being defined by them or overly attached to them. 'Acceptance' is a difficult word for a lot of clients so 'openness', 'willingness' and 'allowing' may be preferred. However, we are still describing an active embrace rather than a passive resignation.

SELF AS CONTEXT

Throughout the sessions, clients are encouraged to recognise that they are not the story they tell themselves about themselves. The concept of the observing self (pure aware-ness) is a helpful one to create some distance between the client and their experiences, particularly when there is a dominant negative self-narrative. This is central to Polk's Psychological Flexibility Matrix (Polk & Schoendorff, 2014; see Figure 6.2), and I often explain that this is a safe place to come back to. Clients often get that those moments when they feel most connected to themselves (and when they have had some respite from the mind's incessant internal monologue) is when they feel at one with their experiencing and their environment.

DEFUSION

Defusion is used to describe the opposite of being fused with our own thoughts. Being able to recognise and distance yourself from thoughts allows them to have much less impact upon you in that moment. This can also be described as a meta-cognitive skill. When we are in a fused state, we completely buy into and believe our thoughts as facts, and we are much more likely to be reactive to events as and when they occur. When we can learn to create space between ourselves and our thinking, and not exclusively pay attention to this process, we are more able to make choices based on what we care about.

Process issues are addressed throughout therapy as the intervention is essentially a Functional Analytic approach to therapy. In that case, we are interested in spotting and naming Antecedents, Behaviours and Consequences as and when they arise in the therapy session. For example, 'I noticed just then that you seemed to get hooked by that thought the mind gave to you about the type of person your mum thinks you should be, I wonder how that thought is working for you? Does it take you closer to the life you want or further away?'

TOP TIPS

Establish Values, explaining early on in the session that the focus of therapeutic work can be about helping clients to move towards a life that they want to build for themselves based upon their own Values: 'How do you become the architect of your own life?'

Establish workability as a criterion by asking: 'How is doing what you are doing now working for you in your life? Is it taking you closer to the life you want or further away?'

Establish the normality of Experiential Avoidance in humans: 'Understandably we do not like experiencing difficult thoughts, feelings, bodily sensations and memories. If there was a way to remove all the painful stuff in my life, I would want that too.' Recognise that this is present in the therapy room for us as well as our clients.

STORIES FROM PRACTICE

Challenging internalised stigmas and self-perceptions

Harry, aged 70, came to therapy following many years of psychiatric care. He had previously refused the offer of psychological therapy on several occasions for fear that it might entail

(Continued)

'digging up the past'. His wife and two daughters felt that his mental health had compromised his family life and his career as he would often physically run away when things got difficult. During our first session Harry gave an in-depth and insightful account of the way in which his 'mental illness' had affected him. I explained that not everyone believed in psychiatric labels or found them to be helpful. Following the assessment and psychoeducation sessions, a case conceptualisation of his difficulties, based on what he had told me, was shared. Harry had spent many years pathologising his thoughts, feelings and behaviour. He viewed his lapses into psychosis as 'some form of defect' and evidence of 'broken genes'. We spent time in the early sessions really clarifying what mattered to him in the here and now, and what he wanted the rest of his life to be about. He was able to recognise that his self-concept was as 'a psychiatric patient'. As a result, all of his experiences were viewed as 'not normal' or 'not valid' and interpreted as symptoms of a disease rather than simply part of his past programming and understandable reactions to feeling quite threatened and overwhelmed at times in his life.

The use of short-term fixes perpetuated his experiential avoidance through medication, over-thinking and intellectualising. Attempting to problem-solve all of these things had not taken him closer to a solution, but taken him further away from what mattered in his life. Harry was able to see that his self-concept over many years had kept him stuck and unable to move forward in his life for fear of the mind's suggestions about 'becoming unwell'. He was also able to see that the things he found painful and the things that he valued were two sides of the same coin. At the end of our brief work together Harry signed up for a local Mindfulness course and made several commitments to continue the progress he had made in our 14 sessions together, including finding a bolt hole that he could escape to when he felt overwhelmed by life or needed space.

Working with teenage peer relationships and social anxieties, clarifying values and defusing unhelpful thoughts about self and others

Shannon, aged 14, was referred with adjustment difficulties following a serious health scare that resulted in several days of hospitalisation in intensive care. Her parents and older siblings were worried about the impact this was having on her and her school work as she had frequently refused to go to school and was often very distressed by things that had been said to her by her school friends. An assessment with her revealed that there were social issues in and outside the school environment that were contributing to anxiety about relationships with her peers and that this in fact was what was currently affecting her more than the initial referral regarding the unexpected illness.

We called the sessions 'Life Skills' as a way of acknowledging that these were simply things that she needed to develop rather than any suggestion that something was 'wrong with her'. A mini formulation was developed to help her understand the impact of her thoughts and feelings on her behaviour and how she was currently struggling to be herself in her peer relationships because she was frightened by her own judgements of herself and what others were thinking of her. We used the DNA-V model, which is a developmental approach to ACT developed by Louise Hayes and Joseph Ciarrochi (2015). Introducing Shannon to the three different parts of herself, the Discoverer, the Advisor and the Noticer, and being able to move flexibly between these different parts of herself helped her to recognise the cost of taking too much notice of the Advisor at times when the Noticer or Discoverer might be more helpful.

We also met with her parents to examine their reactions to some of the things that were happening to Shannon. They admitted that due to their stress levels and over-concern about their daughter's health they tended to be reactive to any perceived threats, such as her peers leaving her out from social occasions or school being hard on her for not completing homework. We discussed how easy it was for them to be bullied by their own thoughts and feelings rather than allowing their values and the longer-term picture to be a priority. For example, they valued their daughter having friends and close confiding relationships and recognised that they wanted to be supportive throughout the ups and downs of school life without resorting to moving schools or complaining to the head each week. They could also understand that instilling in Shannon a belief in her own ability to work through such things in the longer term would be a hugely important life skill. Shannon had 16 sessions.

The longer-term impact of acquired brain injury and its effects on the conceptualised self

Clare was a 37-year-old mother of three young children who had experienced a stroke five years previously. It had taken her a long time to recover from this event and she was unable to return to her previous level of functioning as a consequence. Clare was referred to me by her case manager. She had remained involved in her care over the years after her discharge from the acute rehabilitation setting. Clare reported that she had always had 'social anxiety and depression' since the stroke.

We spent the first few sessions focused on Values and what Clare wanted her life to be like. A lot of the views she had of herself were based on unhelpful comparisons of where she felt she would be now if the stroke hadn't taken place. We spent some time looking at the impact of such an acquired brain injury, but we also spent time and sessions on understanding the threat system and the way in which this could be easily activated when Clare felt overwhelmed and tired or compared herself unfavourably to her mind's generation of the ideal self. Acceptance and self-compassion formed the main basis for our work. Clare, like other clients I have worked with, took great relief in the psychoeducation and facts about the brain and how it worked – 'It's actually normal to feel anxious?' – understanding that her experiences weren't related to this fused idea of a 'broken brain' and that her description of the situations that caused anxiety were more a sign that her brain was working perfectly well. It was also helpful for her to understand that this was the default position for lots of people, that social situations can be tricky to work out and that this only improved with practice, just like learning other skills. We used a lot of compassionate Mindfulness-based exercises and experiential exercises (loving kindness, band of light and healing hand) for Clare to get a felt sense of what the alternative approach to treating herself would look like. She was encouraged to recognise when she became hooked by certain stories that her mind presented to her, such as the 'Oh, I'm not able to cope with this because I have a brain injury' story, when in fact lots of other people without brain injury might find the very same situation difficult or tiring. We also used lots of visual prompts around her home to remind her of the things that mattered to her. For example, Clare produced an image that was important to her – of her and her family in a place they had always loved to visit – and she typed onto the image all of the qualities that mattered to her as a mother and as a person to help her reconnect when she was struggling with her own strong emotions. We also produced other cue cards, giving her prompts to

(Continued)

follow so that she could reconnect with the present moment when she might feel swept away with strong thoughts or feelings. Clare could carry these with her and strategically put them around the house to remind her of them. Clare worked with me for 12 sessions of therapy and a further six sessions of monthly follow-ups.

The role of the Observing Self and Mindfulness to bring about greater internal harmony

Julie was a 32-year-old trainee nurse who had experienced a psychotic breakdown several years earlier following several stressful life events that had coincided. She came to see me during her training as she felt extremely stressed on her placement. Following on from the psychoeducation, we used lots of experiential exercises in therapy to help her to defuse from the thoughts about herself around being 'weak' and feeling frightened of any sensations in her body. Distressing thoughts that she couldn't control or rationalise or simply feeling exhausted, and any sensation or pain in her body or when feeling annoyed or angry at her partner or colleagues, would then lead to tremendous guilt and self-doubt. Julie recognised that she spent a lot of time lost in her own mind, trying to problem solve and evaluate how she had ended up having the breakdown. As a consequence, this was more tiring for her and she recognised that she was very rarely in the present moment.

Julie admitted that she constantly put pressure on herself to be more professional or a better mother and to control the anxiety and other difficult emotions she felt when around colleagues, patients and family. Julie was encouraged to use various Mindfulness practices throughout her day in work to ground herself in the present, and this enabled her to get out of her mind and into the here and now, using her senses and her breathing. We used the matrix diagram as a ready reckoner for her to continually come back to and to recognise when she was lost in her mind versus coming back to this grounded perspective of the Observing Self. Julie was able to see that she had tended to cut herself off from feeling difficult emotions or would berate herself for having them, and we spent time focused upon an exposure-based approach to her negative emotions.

In essence, Julie was able to understand, by using an adapted version of the stress vulnerability bucket, that the psychotic breakdown she had was as a result of having very little capacity over many years and this finally tipping over. Julie understood that what she had learnt through our sessions was a way of building her resilience to enable her to do the career she loved and to pursue the life she wanted with her family, but that there was no way of achieving this without acceptance of the difficult thoughts, feelings and bodily sensations that naturally and normally show up. Julie worked with me for eight sessions, but our work was limited by the lack of funding from her employer.

Using the Observing Self and Mindfulness to unhook from habitual unhelpful thinking patterns

Terence, a local farmer, had been increasingly distressed due to the arrival of his third child and financial fears involving his business. He was reluctant to seek therapy as, in the farming community, 'mental illness' still carried the taboo of the old inpatient hospital days. During the early stages of assessment and psychoeducation, Terence repeatedly asserted that he did not know how this (talking) was helping him. Despite this, he booked and attended subsequent appointments. By his own admission, Terence spent a lot of time focused on the worst-case scenario and what might go wrong in any given situation. As a consequence, his generalised worry and procrastination were being managed by the people around him, with family and colleagues walking on eggshells or not asking him to do things for fear of his reaction.

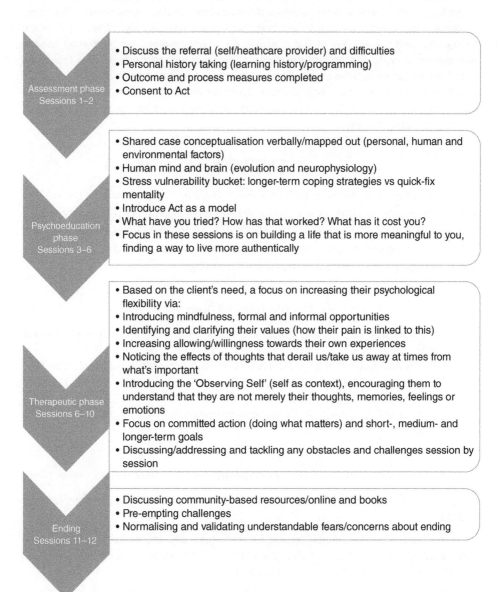

Assessment phase
Sessions 1–2
- Discuss the referral (self/heathcare provider) and difficulties
- Personal history taking (learning history/programming)
- Outcome and process measures completed
- Consent to Act

Psychoeducation phase
Sessions 3–6
- Shared case conceptualisation verbally/mapped out (personal, human and environmental factors)
- Human mind and brain (evolution and neurophysiology)
- Stress vulnerability bucket: longer-term coping strategies vs quick-fix mentality
- Introduce Act as a model
- What have you tried? How has that worked? What has it cost you?
- Focus in these sessions is on building a life that is more meaningful to you, finding a way to live more authentically

Therapeutic phase
Sessions 6–10
- Based on the client's need, a focus on increasing their psychological flexibility via:
- Introducing mindfulness, formal and informal opportunities
- Identifying and clarifying their values (how their pain is linked to this)
- Increasing allowing/willingness towards their own experiences
- Noticing the effects of thoughts that derail us/take us away at times from what's important
- Introducing the 'Observing Self' (self as context), encouraging them to understand that they are not merely their thoughts, memories, feelings or emotions
- Focus on committed action (doing what matters) and short-, medium- and longer-term goals
- Discussing/addressing and tackling any obstacles and challenges session by session

Ending
Sessions 11–12
- Discussing community-based resources/online and books
- Pre-empting challenges
- Normalising and validating understandable fears/concerns about ending

Figure 6.5 Flowchart illustrating the general approach taken for clients with mild–moderate mental health difficulties using ACT

We focused heavily on developing everyday informal as well as more formal Mindfulness skills as well as clarifying his core values. He was introduced to the idea of engaging with Mindfulness in the same way he would with other daily habits – brushing twice a day prevents tooth decay. You don't wait until you need root canal surgery to start brushing! Several sessions into therapy, Terence came in and asserted 'I get it now'. He had begun to understand more about his typical reaction to things and that there was an alternative viewpoint.

We use the term 'wiggle room' to define the space that can develop during creative hopelessness, when clients are able to see that there is not just one way of seeing or doing things. We used the analogy of the stream and the embankment, which is often used in Mindfulness work, to encapsulate the Observer Self that he could access: even though he may fall into the stream numerous times a day, there was an alternative place where he could get out of the water and onto dry land. Terence worked with me for 14 sessions before opting to start a local initiative bringing isolated farmers together to benefit from 'Life Skills' such as Mindfulness.

CONCLUSION

ACT is an approach to working with two issues. The first is what makes us human and how we can create suffering for ourselves in our attempts to get rid of pain from our lives. The second is how pain, emotional or physical, is an inevitable part of life. Pain and values are two sides of the same coin. Anything you care about can lead to painful experiences, but this is not necessarily a symptom of pathology.

DISCUSSION QUESTIONS

1. What are the distinct processes that differ between generic CBT and ACT as a third-wave model?
2. How does ACT differ from other models that focus on Acceptance and Mindfulness?
3. What are some of the considerations that you as a therapist might take into account when introducing ACT to a client?
4. How would working from an ACT philosophy change or influence you as a person or as a clinician?

KEY TERMS

Acceptance and Commitment Therapy (ACT) A third-wave transdiagnostic psychotherapeutic approach.

ACT home practice An invitation to practise techniques and approaches explored in sessions, putting decisions and actions into place in the client's 'real world' to test feasibility and impact. This term is used instead of the term 'homework'.

Behaviour Analysis A science based on the foundations of Behaviourism.

Dialectical Behavioural Therapy (DBT) This was developed as a psychological approach to working with clients labelled as having a Borderline Personality Disorder and clients who were chronically suicidal.

Functional Analytic Psychotherapy (FAP) An approach to therapy based on radical Behaviourism.

Hexaflex Model A model that illustrates the core concepts of Acceptance and Commitment Therapy and how they interrelate.

Mindfulness-Based Cognitive Therapy (MBCT) An approach to psychotherapy that incorporates mindfulness and mindful awareness of throught and emotions, originally created as a relapse-prevention treatment for depression.

Mindfulness-Based Stress Reduction (MBSR) An eight-week programme based on Mindfulness, meditation and yoga that was initially developed in the area of chronic pain and is now used for a range of clinical and non-clinical problems.

Psychological flexibility In everyday language, this is the ability to pursue your values and the things that make life meaningful while holding your own internal experiences (thoughts, feelings, bodily sensations and memories) lightly.

Relational Frame Theory (RFT) A psychological theory of human language that explains the relationship between higher cognitive functions and language use; also called linguistic determinism.

Transdiagnostic (applies to more than one condition) An approach to understanding psychological distress that is outside the conceptual notion of diagnostic categories.

Valued Living Questionnaire (VLQ) A means of assessing the 10 most valued domains of living.

FURTHER READING

- Harris, R., & Aisbett, B. (2014). *The happiness trap pocketbook*. London: Robinson. Popular myths about happiness directly contribute to our epidemic of stress, anxiety and depression – and some popular remedies are making it even worse! In his original bestselling self-help book, Dr Russ Harris revealed how millions of people are unwittingly caught in 'The Happiness Trap'. He then provides an effective means to escape: ACT (or Acceptance and Commitment Therapy) is based on the principles of Mindfulness.
- Sinclair, M., & Beadman, M. (2016). *The little ACT workbook: An introduction to acceptance and commitment therapy: A mindfulnessbased guide for leading a full and meaningful life*. Bath, UK: Crimson Publishing. A practical introduction to Acceptance and Commitment Therapy (ACT) for the general reader. It is a simple, hands-on, practical guide introducing essential ACT techniques that you can use to live a full and meaningful life and change your life for the better.
- Hayes, S. C., Strosahl, K. D., & Wilson, K. G. (2011). *Acceptance and Commitment Therapy: The process and practice of mindful change* (2nd ed.). New York: Guilford Press. Since the original publication of this seminal work (Hayes et al., 1999), Acceptance and Commitment Therapy has come into its own as a widely practised approach to helping people change. This book provides the definitive statement of ACT – from its conceptual and empirical foundations to clinical techniques – written by its originators.
- Zettle, R. D. (2005). The evolution of a contextual approach to therapy: From Comprehensive Distancing to ACT. *International Journal of Behavioural and Consultation*

Therapy, 1(2), 77-89. An exploration of the developmental history of Acceptance and Commitment Therapy, with recommendations for research and practice.

- Hayes, S. C. (2004). Acceptance and Commitment Therapy and the new behaviour therapies: Mindfulness, acceptance and relationship. In S. C. Hayes, V. M. Follette, & M. Linehan (Eds.), *Mindfulness and acceptance: Expanding the cognitive behavioural tradition* (pp. 1-29). New York: Guilford Press. A critical consideration of the impact of such approaches upon the conceptualisations of behaviour and behaviour change.
- Hayes, S. C., Luoma, J. B., Bond, F. W., Masuda, A. and Lillis, J. (2006). Acceptance and commitment therapy: Model, processes, and outcomes. *Behaviour Research and Therapy,* 44, 1-25.

ONLINE RESOURCES

- The Association for Contextual Behavioural Science (ACBS): https://contextualscience. org
- The Association for Behavioural and Cognitive Therapies (ABCT): www.abct.org/Informa tion/?m=mInformation&fa=CBT_News_sub_02
- The British Association for Behavioural and Cognitive Psychotherapies (BABCP): www. babcp.com/Default.aspx
- The Valued Living Questionnaire (Wilson et al., 2010): https://div12.org/wp-content/ uploads/2015/06/Valued-Living-Questionnaire.pdf
- Acceptance and Action Questionnaire (AAQ-II, Bond et al., 2011): http://integrativehealth-partners.org/downloads/ACTmeasures.pdf
- Mindful Attention Awareness Scale (Brown & Ryan, 2003): https://ppc.sas.upenn.edu/ resources/questionnaires-researchers/mindful-attention-awareness-scale

REFERENCES

Bach, P., & Hayes S. C. (2002). The use of acceptance and commitment therapy to prevent the rehospitalization of psychotic patients: A randomized controlled trial. *Journal of Consulting and Clinical Psychology, 70,* 1129–1139.

Bond, F. W., Hayes, S. C., Baer, R. A., Carpenter, K. M., Guenole, N., Orcutt, H. K., Waltz, T., & Zettle, R. D. (2011). Preliminary psychometric properties of the Acceptance and Action Questionnaire – II: A revised measure of psychological flexibility and experiential avoidance. *Behavior Therapy, 42,* 676–688.

Brown, K. W., & Ryan, R. M. (2003). The benefits of being present: Mindfulness and its role in psychological well-being. *Journal of Personality and Social Psychology, 84,* 822–848.

Cartwright, J., & Hooper, N. (2017). Evaluating a transdiagnostic acceptance and commitment therapy psychoeducation intervention. *The Cognitive Behaviour Therapist, 10*(e9), 1–6. Available from: http://eprints.uwe.ac.uk/33055

Flaxman, P., Bond, F., & Livheim, F. (2013). *Mindful and effective employees: A training program for maximizing well-being and effectiveness using acceptance and commitment therapy.* London: New Harbinger.

Forman, E. M., Herbert, J. D., Moitra, E., Yeomans, P. D., & Geller, P. A. (2007). A randomized controlled effectiveness trial of acceptance and commitment therapy and cognitive therapy for anxiety and depression. *Behavior Modification, 31*(6), 772–799.

Gregg, J., Callaghan, G., & Hayes, S. C. (2007). *The diabetes lifestyle book: Facing your fears and making changes for a long and healthy life.* Oakland, CA: New Harbinger.

Harris, R., & Aisbett, B. (2014). *The happiness trap pocketbook.* London: Robinson.

Hayes, L., & Ciarrochi, J. (2015). *The thriving adolescent: Using acceptance and commitment therapy and positive psychology to help teens manage emotions, achieve goals, and build connections.* Oakland, CA: Context Press/New Harbinger.

Hayes, S. C. (2009). *Acceptance & Commitment Therapy (ACT).* Available from: https://contextualscience.org/act (accessed 10 September 2017).

Hayes, S. C., Barnes-Holmes, D., & Roche, B. (Eds.). (2001). *Relational Frame Theory: A post-Skinnerian account of human language and cognition.* New York: Plenum Press.

Hayes, S. C., Strosahl, K. D., & Wilson, K., G. (1999). *Acceptance and Commitment Therapy: An experiential approach to behaviour change.* New York: Guilford Press. Available from: http://thehappinesstrap.com/upimages/the_house_of Act (accessed 10 September 2017).

McCracken, L. M., & Vowles, K. E. (2014). Acceptance and commitment therapy and mindfulness for chronic pain: Model, process, and progress. *The American Psychologist, 69*(2), 178–187.

Meadows, G. (2014). *The sleep book: How to sleep well every night.* London: Orion Publishing.

Polk, K. L., & Schoendorff, B. (Eds.). (2014). *The ACT matrix: A new approach to building psychological flexibility across settings and populations.* Oakland, CA: Context Press/New Harbinger.

Rhodes, E. (2014). Commit and ACT on Ebola. *The Psychologist, 27.*

Sahdra, B. K., Ciarrochi, J., & Parker, P. D. (2016). Non-attachment and mindfulness: Related but distinct constructs. *American Psychological Association, 28*(7), 819–829.

Sinclair, M., & Beadman, M. (2016). *The little ACT workbook.* Bath, UK: Crimson Publishing.

Strosahl, K., Robinson, P., & Gustavsson, T. (2012). *Brief interventions for radical change: Principles and practice of focused acceptance and commitment therapy.* Oakland, CA: New Harbinger.

Vowles, K. E., Wetherell, J. L., & Sorrell, J. T. (2009). Targeting acceptance, mindfulness, and values-based action in chronic pain: Findings of two preliminary trials of an outpatient group-based intervention. *Cognitive and Behavioral Practice, 16,* 49–58.

Wilson, K. G., Sandoz, E. K., Kitchens, J., & Roberts, M. E. (2010). The Valued Living Questionnaire: Defining and measuring valued action within a behavioral framework. *The Psychological Record, 60,* 249–272.

7

BRIEF DYNAMIC INTERPERSONAL THERAPY

CATHERINE ATHANASIADOU-LEWIS AND VENETIA LEONIDAKI

INTRODUCTION

This chapter will discuss the development of Dynamic Interpersonal Therapy (DIT), a brief psychodynamic model, designed for the treatment of depression and anxiety (Lemma, Target, & Fonagy, 2011a). The aim of this chapter is to:

- navigate our readers through the main theoretical origins of DIT by offering a historical overview of the development of brief psychodynamic therapy
- familiarise you with the specific methods and techniques of DIT by outlining the model's technical and process features *vis-à-vis* an evidence-based activity
- offer a real-life perspective of DIT's characteristics in practice by discussing case material and evaluating the model's position within the psychodynamic paradigm.

HISTORICAL OVERVIEW OF THE ORIGINS OF BRIEF PSYCHODYNAMIC THERAPY

At first glance, the terms 'brief' and 'psychodynamic' may read as an oxymoron. But when combined together, they refer to a structured and systematic therapeutic approach to mental health difficulties. Derived from psychoanalysis, psychodynamic therapy is traditionally associated with long-term analytic work, which focuses on the exploration and interpretation of unconscious intrapsychic and interpersonal phenomena, with an aim to achieve personality change through insight and psycho-structural transformation (Fenichel, 1996). At the centre of psychoanalytic theory is the concept of the 'dynamic unconscious': the component of the human mind that hosts conflictual emotional forces in constant relation to each other, and which determines to a large extent all human motivation, cognition, affect and behaviour. While the dynamic unconscious operates outside one's awareness, its contents (such as memories, feelings or mental representations) can be accessed through the careful analysis of a person's unintentional behaviours, actions, discourses and dreams.

Freud chose the term 'dynamic' (Greek δύναμαι = to have force) in relation to the unconscious because he observed that the internal changes that endure within us may be the result of psychic 'energy' (Greek ενέργεια = internal work) owing to the operation of incompatible instinctual forces, such as aggression and libido. In his structural model, Freud referred to the oppositional nature of these forces as 'intrapsychic conflict' – the Id's wish for sexual gratification from a significant other, for example, may come into conflict with the Superego's ethical codes, resulting in feelings of anxiety that the Ego will then need to regulate according to its strength (Freud, 1923).

Studying clinical material from patients (see *Studies on hysteria*, Breuer & Freud, 1895) and analysing his own dreams, Freud came to hypothesise that much of mental life is instinctually motivated, but he also went on to elaborate the importance of childhood experiences in shaping human personality; the operation of intrapsychic defence mechanisms (e.g. projection, repression) designed to relieve the individual from debilitating angst by avoiding distressing affects; and the significance of symbolism in interpersonal communication, relational depiction and symptom formation (Fenichel, 1996).

Freud viewed symbolism (Greek συμβάλλειν = thrown together) as a sign of the indirect expression of an impetus, and assigned to symbolic behaviour a defensive function, in terms of 'unconsciously producing a substitute' (Petosz, 1999, p. 14) for something that has been repressed, for example, a wish, a conflict or a forbidden phantasy. As a result, Freud was concerned with the metaphorical parallels between a patient's symptom (e.g. self-harming in depression) and their original yet 'forbidden' aim (e.g. a wish to attack an internalised part of the ego).

Of utmost analytic importance was the clinical observation that humans tend to repeat earlier patterns of relating in an attempt to master a conflict arising from an earlier repressed, traumatic or otherwise hurtful experience. Freud captured this phenomenon in his early writings on 'remembering, repeating and working through' and termed it 'compulsion to repeat' (Freud, 1914, p. 151). Attending to his patients' relational patterns using free association, Freud discovered the notion of transference, a relational phenomenon whereby the therapist (and other important people) may symbolically represent a figure from the patient's past. By closely attending to the manifestations of the transference (e.g. how the patient treats the therapist, their expectations, wishes and anticipated roles) and gradually interpreting its aim (e.g. a wish to dominate a controlling parent by overpowering the therapist), Freud was the first clinician who attributed therapeutic change to the powers of the therapeutic relationship – albeit in a positivist manner, where the analyst acted as an 'observer' as opposed to an 'active participant' in the therapeutic process (Halewood, 2017).

While classical psychoanalysis relies on long-term work with regular weekly sessions, Freud's original psychoanalysis varied. For example, Freud wrote extensively about Dora's analysis, which ended prematurely at 11 weeks, or his encounter with the case of Katharina, where he had to provide a brief consultation on what we now know as panic attacks, during his vacation. In 1937, Freud experimented with setting a definite ending date during analysis with a Russian man whose progress had stalled, and explored the value of planned endings in accelerating the dismantling of patients' resistances.

The evolution of psychoanalytic theory gradually transitioned into the development of psychodynamic theory, encompassing further revisions to Freud's original formulations, including Jung's analytical psychology, the school of Object Relations (Melanie Klein, Donald Winnicott, Ronald Fairbairn, John Bowlby), interpersonal psychoanalysis (Harry Stack Sullivan, Erich Fromm) and the school of self-psychology (Heinz Kohut), to name a few. Followers of Freud, such as Klein, Winnicott and Bion, developed his original model further and included the realm of human object relating, that is, the centrality of relationships, particularly attachment processes and infancy experiences, in the formation of personality and 'character pathology'. Collectively, Object Relations theorists centred on the idea that the individual is motivated by the need for relationships; drives such as aggression and sexuality were conceptualised as operating *within relationships* rather than *within the person* (Halewood, 2017). Gradually, clinical practice shifted from the '*sole individual*' to the '*individual that is in need for other*' (Lemma et al., 2011a, p. 36). Halewood (2017) refers to this transition as the shift from a 'one-person psychology' to the 'two-persons relational perspective', and it shaped contemporary psychodynamic practice, with its emphasis on mutuality, intersubjectivity and the therapist's inevitable involvement in the relationship.

> The idea that both therapist and client contributed to, and were affected by, the relational dynamics gained increasing acceptance leading to a move away from the hierarchical towards a recognition of the mutual. (Halewood, 2017, p. 94)

The advancement of the psychodynamic approach saw changes both in its ontological positions, in terms of assuming an investment in the relational paradigm, as briefly outlined above, and in terms of technique, orientation and resources. So, from the modernist years of Darwin and Freud all the way to postwar and postmodernist Britain and Western civilisation in general, the growth of psychotherapy has been marked by the neoliberal scene of a state invested in undoing social harm (Barr, 2004). Therapeutic provision within public health meant a turn towards science and practice (namely the evidence-base model), with a healthcare mentality that alluded to resources as much as it aspired to psychic healing. Gradually, brief psychodynamic therapy gained momentum, with Michael Balint and David Malan being the first psychoanalysts to propose a measurable, short-term version of psychodynamic therapy that would centre around a clinical 'focus', retaining the basic tools of interpretation and transference, but sacrificing other techniques, such as therapeutic passivity, open-endedness and character transformation (Mander, 2000). The growing body of research supporting the efficacy of short-term models (for a full review, see Abbas et al., 2014) and their technical emphasis on generating more rapid therapeutic results, as compared to the classical open-ended psychoanalytic approach, have made brief psychodynamic therapy an attractive treatment option for certain mental health conditions in public health – precisely because cost-effectiveness is a key factor in the National Health Service (NHS). Indeed, irrespective of the specific theoretical model, short-term psychodynamic therapies preserve essential elements of psychoanalytic therapy, such as the focus on affective and relational themes, the exploration of defences and past experiences, and an emphasis on the therapeutic relationship, wishes and fantasies (Shedler, 2010). These defining elements set apart psychodynamic therapy from other treatment approaches, such as cognitive behavioural therapy (CBT). In the following section, we focus specifically on a certain kind of brief psychodynamic therapy, Dynamic Interpersonal Therapy (DIT), which has maintained the distinct elements of psychodynamic therapy mentioned above, but has been adapted specifically for the treatment of depression within the NHS in England.

BACKGROUND TO THE DEVELOPMENT OF DIT

DIT can be seen as the 'socio-analytical child' of the evidence-based era, as it arose in the context of the Improving Access to Psychological Therapies (IAPT) programme in the NHS in England (Care Services Improvement Partnership, 2007). The success of IAPT relied on the delivery of evidence-based psychological therapies by a large workforce of clinically competent therapists. In particular, DIT was developed hand in hand with two series of documents: the *Competencies Framework*, outlining the competencies that psychological therapists need to have to practise in certain treatment modalities, and the *National Occupational Standards*, describing the performance required of individuals in their workplace (Roth & Pilling, 2007). Originating in the psychoanalytic/psychodynamic tradition, DIT has a very different focus from other psychological interventions in IAPT and, as a result, satisfies the need for making available a range of therapies for depression.

DIT: THEORETICAL UNDERPINNINGS AND CORE FEATURES

The core principles of DIT are embedded in the Object Relations school, the concepts of attachment and mentalisation, and Sullivan's interpersonal theory (Lemma et al., 2011a). As discussed in the introductory section, the term 'Object Relations' covers a range of theories, which share an emphasis on an inner world consisting of mental representations of self and others (Glickauf-Hughes & Wells, 1997). Early interactions with primary caregivers play a crucial role in the quality of one's internal objects and in shaping a person's character. Essentially, internal objects significantly affect one's way of relating to others. These theories highlight the fundamental need for the caregiver to help the infant manage primitive anxieties by metabolising raw emotional material to a more processed and easily-digested experience (Gomez, 1997). DIT focuses on the way that interpersonal functioning in depression is influenced by the impact of internalised, unconscious representations of self and others.

The next major theoretical framework of DIT is Attachment Theory (Bowlby, 1969/1982). Influenced by Object Relations, Bowlby (1969/1982) developed the concept of Internal Working Models (IWM) to describe the representational models of others and self, stemming from early interactions with the caregiver. Thus, the quality of early attachments plays a tremendous role in various domains of psychosocial development, such as peer relationships (Allen, Moore, Kuperminc, & Bell, 1998), affect regulation (Spangler & Zimmermann, 1999) and self-concept (Wu, 2009).

Following the above line of thinking, Fonagy, Steele, Moran, Steele, and Higgitt (1991) drew connections between attachment processes and reflective functioning. Further, Fonagy and Target (1997) introduced the term 'mentalisation' to describe one's ability to understand mental states in self and others (e.g. thoughts, feelings, intentions, wishes) and developed a model relating to insufficient mentalising capacity, which originates in the caregiver's difficulty in understanding the infant's mental states and communicating them back to the child, to a pathological self. According to this model, the main therapeutic goal is enhancing patients' mentalising capacity (Fonagy, Gergely, Jurist, & Target, 2002).

DIT has also drawn ideas from interpersonal psychoanalysis. Sullivan (1953) placed human behaviour in the wider interpersonal and social context as he believed in a constant dialogue between the inner mental events (e.g. how one imagines others to be) and the external reality of interpersonal experiences (e.g. how others actually are). He viewed the need to minimise insecurity as the main motivational force, even though this would sometimes inadvertently lead to distress and relationships damaging to one's self-esteem.

Having drawn from the above theoretical ideas, DIT understands the symptoms of depression and anxiety in mainly interpersonal terms. More specifically, when certain individuals perceive external/internal triggers as threatening to their attachments and sense of self, such as a significant loss, they tend to respond with distortions in thinking and feelings typical of depression (e.g. excessive criticism and guilt) and anxiety. Various psychological processes are involved in these responses. DIT recognises the importance of unconscious forces and intrapersonal conflicts, as outlined earlier. However, its emphasis is on how difficult early experiences and insecure attachments (represented as negative IWMs of self and others) influence interpersonal functioning and play a predisposing role in depression in later life (Lemma et al., 2011a). This position is in line with a growing body of evidence that links insecure attachments to depression (e.g. Blatt & Homman, 1992; Burnette, Davis, Green, Worthington, & Bradfield, 2009) and highlights the mediating role of low self-esteem (e.g. Roberts, Gotlib, & Kassel, 1996). Closely linked to insecure attachments and negative IWMs are an impaired reflective capacity and failures of mentalisation (Fonagy & Target, 1997). In depression, these difficulties in mentalisation present themselves in two different ways: either as concrete thinking, reflected in complaints about bodily instead of psychological experiences, or in pseudo-mentalising, where thinking about the mental states of oneself and others takes place but in a repetitive and excessively detailed manner that reinforces individuals' negative perspectives (e.g. rumination; Lemma et al., 2011a).

EVIDENCE-BASED ACTIVITY

Relevant effectiveness research on DIT to date has been limited to small studies (Lemma, Target, & Fonagy, 2011b). In the first study (n=14), 87.5% of participants completed the whole course of DIT and almost 70% of the participants scored at or below the clinical cut-off for depression and anxiety at the end of therapy. The reduction in symptoms appeared significant, with the fastest reduction happening in the first few sessions. In the second study, 42% improved reliably for anxiety and 25% for depression (Wright & Abrahams, 2015). Both studies were uncontrolled, so the significance cannot be reliably attributed to DIT, while their small sample size provides only preliminary evidence for its effectiveness. There are currently two randomised evaluations of DIT taking place. The first study compares the outcomes of participants diagnosed with depression who are receiving DIT with participants on the enhanced waiting list who have contact with a psychological wellbeing practitioner once a fortnight. The second study is a feasibility study that paves the way for a larger trial of DIT; it compares the outcomes of 40 adults with depression who receive DIT with a group who receive CBT. To date, no results for these two studies have been published (www.redit.org.uk/why.php).

TOP TIP

To develop a good Interpersonal-Affective Focus, attend to one repetitive theme relevant to the client's interpersonal style (e.g. relying on self-sufficiency and avoiding asserting needs to others, leading the client to feel like a burden and imagine others to be dismissive). This focus will capture the conscious affect that connects the two: e.g. anger about becoming ignored. A foundation is then laid to explore the preconscious affect that is subtler and to help the client own and process it: e.g. despair about being worthless and unimportant to others; fantasy of extinction if needs remain ungratified.

DIT IN CLINICAL PRACTICE: ITS CORE FEATURES

Lemma et al. (2011a) explain that DIT has two primary aims:

1. To help the patient understand the connection between his presenting symptoms and his current relationships, through identifying a core, unconscious pattern of relating, that is repetitive throughout his life and becomes the focus of therapy.
2. To encourage the patient to reflect on his own states of mind and so strengthen his ability to deal with interpersonal difficulties. (Lemma et al., 2011a, p. 63)

AN ACTIVE ANALYTIC STANCE

In DIT, the stance is an analytic one in the sense that the therapist keeps an anonymous and neutral stance, shows an interest in the patient's conscious and unconscious communication and favours reflection over action. However, in order to facilitate change in a short amount of time, there is a need for a more active, engaging style than that adopted in long-term analytic work, where long silences are common (Bordne, 1999).

WORKING ON AN INTERPERSONAL-AFFECTIVE FOCUS

DIT is organised around an interpersonal-affective focus (IPAF) that is formulated in the initial phase of therapy. More specifically, the therapist helps the patient to identify a dominant, recurrent, usually preconscious, interpersonal pattern directly linked to their presenting problem. Influenced by Kernberg's (1980) ideas, the IPAF conceptualises mental representations of self (e.g. 'hard to manage' infant) and Other (rejecting mother), which are linked to certain conscious (e.g. anger) and unconscious/preconscious affect (e.g. despair). The defensive configuration of IPAF is also important, and specifically illustrates how defence mechanisms both external (pushing away Other by causing arguments) and internal (denigrating Other) are employed in order to protect the ego by the anxiety that the unconscious affect could cause (e.g. the sense of despair that the longing for Other's love would cause). Identifying the IPAF, which serves as a formulation that guides the subsequent therapeutic encounter, is a crucial moment in therapy. Before setting a verbal contract about the focus of therapy, the therapist needs to negotiate the IPAF with the client and ensure that it is meaningful to them.

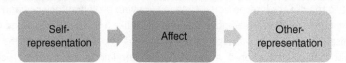

Figure 7.1 IPAF dimensions (Lemma et al., 2011a)
Source: Lemma et al., 2011a

A FOCUS ON THE PATIENT'S MIND

DIT has a consistent emphasis on patients' mental states (beliefs, feelings, wishes and thoughts), both conscious and unconscious, as well as on what mental states clients attribute to others. The therapist shows an interest in the client's mental states, often through asking questions about relationships with others (e.g. 'How did you experience him/her in this situation?') and their connection to the client's own reflections and internal states (e.g. 'How did this make you feel?'). The IPAF also provides a context in which the patient's mentalising capacity can be enhanced by increasing awareness of connections between the patient's behaviour and their conscious and preconscious mental states ('It sounds like you pushed him away because you felt hurt and rejected'). The rationale under-lying this practice is that the patient's experience of thinking with another person about his/her own mental states will enhance his/her reflective capacity (Fonagy et al., 2002).

TOP TIP

To enhance reflective capacity, actively encourage the client to reflect on things as opposed to holding long silences. Rewind to a moment before an identified failure of mentalising, for example, when a client became disproportionately angry following a minor infraction in a friendship.

A HERE-AND-NOW FOCUS

This has three aspects: a focus on the current difficulties; a focus on affect; and a focus on the therapeutic relationship. Regarding the focus on the current difficulties, the emphasis of therapy is on the patient's presenting problems (e.g. difficulties in relationships with colleagues and friends) rather than on early experiences where the current problems origi-nate (e.g. relationship with mother). In relation to the focus on affect, the therapist helps the patient to identify feelings present in sessions, communicate them more effectively and connect them with other aspects of the patient's experience (e.g. 'I noticed how you became tearful for a moment and then you rushed to change the topic'). Finally, the therapist makes use of the immediacy of the therapeutic relationship to demonstrate bet-ter aspects related to the IPAF.

A CLEAR STRUCTURE

DIT has three distinct phases with clear goals in each one: the initial phase (1–4 sessions), the middle phase (5–12 sessions) and the ending phase (13–16 sessions). The 16-session length is consistent with the length of other available psychological interventions in IAPT.

TOP TIP

Consider the use of defences as a way to distort reality and challenge them only if they relate to the IPAF and they interfere with therapeutic progress. DIT does not aspire to the complete dismantling of defences, but rather helps the client to make sense of what they are resisting and what they need to adapt to. For example, an angry client who feels like a burden, sees others as dismissive and avoids asserting himself due to underlying despair may project this despair onto the therapist by making them feel hopeless or rejected. Using the therapeutic relationship, identify the projected affect and help the client to own it within the safety of the relationship.

APPLICATION OF DIT: WHAT DIT LOOKS LIKE IN PRACTICE
INITIAL PHASE

In the initial phase, the DIT therapist focuses on identifying the patient's interpersonal map by eliciting a thorough account of significant relationships (current and past ones) in a variety of settings, paying particular attention to how they may be linked to presenting problems and their development. The aims of this phase include formulating recurring patterns and refining how the patient experiences self and others, and the linking affect. An understanding of these elements will lead to the identification of IPAF, which will be communicated to the patient so a shared focus for the work can be collaboratively negotiated. A good IPAF should be relevant to presenting problems in a meaningful way for the patient, linked to strong affect, applicable to a variety of relationships and should include pithy descriptors, which often rely on the client's own words and metaphors (e.g. self as 'spare part' and others as 'cold'). As part of the initial phase, the DIT therapist is also interested in understanding the patient's attachment style, and administrating Bartholomew and Horowitz's (1991) attachment scale can be used towards this purpose. Finally, the therapist listens out for the 'cautionary tale' (Ogden, 1992), which concerns the patient's underlying anxieties about therapy and may well be linked to IPAF and presenting problems.

MIDDLE PHASE

In this phase, the therapist offers less guidance, encouraging the client to bring material about his/her week and allowing space for any narratives and unconscious dynamics to emerge and be explored. This phase offers the opportunity for understanding further the defence mechanisms, their cost and function, and, if appropriate, helping the client to think about how to start making changes towards his/her goals. The exploration of the transference may also be used as a platform towards this purpose. Yet the therapist is mainly expected to keep an ear out for material shedding more light on IPAF, which he/she repeatedly refers to and refines. Decisions about the exploration and interpretation of transference will also depend on how such interventions will enrich the IPAF or not. The focus remains on the affective and relational elements of the client's narratives, and the therapeutic relationship can be used as a powerful vehicle for change via exploration of the transference.

ENDING PHASE

In DIT we prepare the client for the ending from the outset by setting a clear contract and making frequent references to the ending throughout therapy. Thus, guided by the IPAF, we now try to understand the unconscious meaning that the ending has for this client and how it may activate certain feelings, fantasies and defences which we may want to bring to the client's attention and, if appropriate, challenge. The 'goodbye' letter that we give to the client at (or near) the 13th session aims to capture the IPAF and offers a summary of the process of therapy, the client's progress and therapeutic relationship, and it is presented as a draft so that the client can also alter it. Sharing the 'goodbye' letter with the client often tends to be an emotionally-charged process and the exploration of the feelings that it may bring is an important part of the work in this final phase of DIT. Further, the letter also aims to act like a transitional object (Winnicott, 1960) and help with relapse prevention.

EVALUATION OF DIT

DIT was primarily designed for treating clients with mild to moderate depression in primary care and, as a result, it is mostly suitable for this client group and less suitable for clients with different types of presenting problem or more severe depression. There is a contrast between insight-orientated psychotherapy and supportive psychotherapy, with a client's treatment usually falling somewhere between these two ends of the spectrum. Although DIT combines elements from both insight-orientated and supportive therapies, it makes certain demands on the patient, including having the capacity and willingness to recognise their role in their difficulties, reflecting on the therapeutic relationship and working towards a focus. Some depressed patients may enter therapy needing a more supportive-orientated approach, which mainly helps them to make sense of their feelings, validate the impact of past losses or draw links between past and present experiences, before they are ready to start understanding their own defences and internal patterns in a time-limited framework, as DIT requires. Can brief dynamic interpersonal therapy ever be judged on its own merits? It's hard to answer with certainty, but Freud may have had something to say about that too:

> Hence, from the very beginning, attempts have been made to shorten the course of analysis. Such endeavours required no justification: they could claim to be prompted by the strongest considerations alike of reason and expediency. But it may be that there lurked in them some trace of the impatient contempt with which the medical profession of an earlier day regarded the neuroses, seeing in them the unnecessary results of invisible lesions. (Freud, 1937, p. 373)

─────────────── STORY FROM PRACTICE ───────────────

Oliver

Oliver is a bright, 42-year-old marketing executive, who presented in therapy due to generalised anxiety and depression. From a very young age, Oliver experienced difficulties with reading and writing due to undiagnosed dyslexia, resulting in feelings of confusion and

(Continued)

distress in primary school. Not being able to understand what was going on for him, Oliver expressed these feelings through disruptive behaviour, while many of his classmates and teachers picked on this and humiliated him excessively. His mother was described as over-protective whereas his father held more of a containing quality; both parents were excelling academics and Oliver often felt that he was a disappointment to them both.

Once diagnosed, he was sent to a boarding school, where he shared the better part of his teenage years surrounded by children with severe learning difficulties. He eventually returned to London where he attended college, was reunited with his family and formed short-lived romantic relationships.

The main interpersonal theme surrounding his relationships was a fear of rejection, which led to submissive and compliant behaviours, with an underlying sense of unfulfilment and frequent loss of sexual interest. At work, Oliver seemed to be very well received and valued, but reported persistent episodes of panic associated with work-related rumination: assuming peers are judging and disapproving of him.

Listening out for the 'cautionary tale' in relation to Oliver's previous experiences of receiving help revealed an initial fantasy about being persecuted by a critical therapist who would eventually punish him rather than support him (in the same fashion his parents and teachers failed to stand by him in his formative years). As a result, Oliver would initially present guarded with a reluctance to share the full realm of his experiences and with a tendency to 'disguise' his impending failures. Using DIT's IPAF formulation, we established a 'focus' on Oliver's interpersonal relations associated with anxiety and depression, and mapped the most significant object-relations enactments. Oliver would define himself as oscillating between social façades of 'thoughtfulness and willingfulness' with a less tangible sense of himself as a 'failure in disguise'. Important others would include his girlfriend and colleagues, which would be collectively seen as 'superior, dominant and rejecting'. The most prominent conscious affect that connected the two was anxiety around performance (including sexual performance), which would manifest itself either in avoidance or in manic attempts at perfecting all professional/ intimate endeavours to avoid rejection.

Embarking on the co-construction of preconscious affect meant a deeper but timely elaboration on the enactments of previous relational patterns (experiences of humiliation at school and limited 'holding' at home), which helped us recover memories of bullying and a deeper sense of 'shameful rage' underlying Oliver's persistent anxiety. Rage was not treated as an isolated emotion, but as a multifaceted preconscious affect that held a shameful substrate too. For Oliver, getting in touch with his intense rage against those object representations that triggered it by humiliating him led to a subsequent fantasy that the anger would destroy his much-needed relationships (in the same way, his disruptive behaviour as a child led to his exile to boarding school, depriving him of his family and valued friendships). Finding it hard to mentalise and make sense of the dimensions and potentials of these affects led Oliver to defend against them by adopting a façade of 'willingfulness to please' in order to keep his destructiveness at bay, by avoiding anticipated criticism and activation of 'shameful rage'. The cost of such entropic prohibition was that Oliver hardly allowed himself the opportunity to fully express his authentic needs and feelings to others, resulting in depressive isolation, culminating in years of frustration and unfulfilment.

During the middle phase of treatment, we collaboratively worked on his fearful-avoidant attachment style and encouraged Oliver to mentalise more flexibly about the way others see him in the present, while negating the destructive aspects of expressing 'shameful rage'. Attending to the transference dynamic, the therapist unconsciously adopted a dominant stance and often controlled and guided the sessions excessively in response to a part of Oliver that felt disguised and disengaged – namely, the aggressive part. Once this dynamic was recognised, Oliver could see his contribution in feeling powerless, and gradually began to experiment with subtle expressions of dissatisfaction and anger in the sessions. The therapeutic relationship was instrumental in the sense that the therapist then acted as a secure base, where Oliver would be able to expose his 'shameful rage' and withstand the anxiety of rejection and destructiveness. The therapist then related to Oliver with a 'disinterested concern', as opposed to the critical/punitive attitude Oliver envisaged, particularly during moments of elusiveness or therapeutic impasse (e.g. when Oliver struggled to make progress, appeared guarded or otherwise 'failed' his therapist). Oliver adapted alternative ways of communicating with others as well, including assertiveness and disinhibition. Alongside that, his internal ghosts were confronted and although work *with* the transference was limited, it was nevertheless discreetly enforced. Oliver found the space to process his unsung anger towards some of the pupils and teachers (and his own parents, to an extent) who had humiliated him in the past, instead of re-enacting these patterns with his girlfriend or colleagues at work, by placing himself in the 'victim' position. He developed a new understanding and paradigm where others could be viewed as '*significant, equal and accepting*', with the power imbalance between 'self' and 'other' gradually diminishing, and the connecting affect of anxiety decreasing too.

During the ending phase in the 13th session, Oliver's initial feelings about the ending resembled his anxious anticipation of being sent to boarding school as a way of punishment for his defectiveness and destructive behaviour. This was elucidated further in the 'Goodbye letter', where DIT could be seen as 'a chapter' (Mander, 2000) leading to another; as a brief yet meaningful encounter that could facilitate a transition to a new psychological territory with resourceful gains. Oliver allowed himself the opportunity to express resentment and 'blame' DIT's principles for the end of this chapter without feeling responsible for it and thus relating to it as '*rejection leading to exile*'. Instead, Oliver treated our ending as '*transition to a familiar new*'. His main therapeutic gains included a more flexible ability to mentalise about others, an expanded repertoire of assertive behaviours centring on the expression of disavowed affects, such as anger, and an appreciation of these affective experiences as authentic mental events, as opposed to treating emotions as a threat to his psychological and physical integrity.

CONCLUSION

DIT is an evidence-based, 16-session brief psychodynamic model designed for the treatment of depression in primary care England. It favours a reflective but active analytic stance, adopts an interpersonal formulation with an emphasis on preconscious affect in the present, and enhances mentalisation capacity with a view to minimise perceived threats to the attachment system. DIT consists of three phases. During the initial phase, the therapist maps the client's interpersonal world and collaboratively works with the client to identify a repeated pattern of relating that is linked to the presenting problem. During the middle phase the therapeutic work centres on the agreed focus, encouraging change and challenging potential resistance to change. The ending phase is heralded by a 'Goodbye letter' in session 13, and the last four sessions bring the work to an end (Abrahams, 2017).

─────────────────────── DISCUSSION QUESTIONS ───────────────────────

1. What elements of psychoanalytic and psychodynamic theory has DIT preserved and how are they applied in practice?
2. Using DIT's IPAF formulation, illustrate a recent case of depression you have to work with.
3. What are the benefits and drawbacks of time-limited DIT?

─────────────────────── FURTHER READING ───────────────────────

- Lemma, A., Target, M., & Fonagy, P. (2011a). *Brief dynamic interpersonal therapy: A clinician's guide*. Oxford: Oxford University Press. A practical guide for the implementation of a brief psychodynamic intervention in clinical practice as well as in research protocols. Written by the pioneers of DIT, this book outlines the development and application of the model in a splendid manner that can educate practitioners across the world. It is an excellent primer for trainees as well as experienced psychodynamic therapists.
- Fonagy, P., Gergely, G., Jurist, G., & Target, M. (2002). *Affect regulation, mentalization and the development of the self*. London: Karnac Books. A comprehensive approach to contemporary psychoanalytic practice. Exploring the centrality of mentalisation and attachment processes in human development and psychopathology, this book offers a contemporary psychoanalytic account of treatment pathways based on case material and an in-depth theoretical engagement that DIT practitioners will find very useful.
- Lemma, A. (2003). *Introduction to the practice of psychoanalytic psychotherapy*. Chichester: Wiley & Sons. An accessible introductory guide to the principles of psychoanalysis. This book is a thorough and comprehensive introduction to the basic theoretical concepts of psychoanalysis, its techniques and associated practice issues. It is ideal for trainees and beginners. It's a skilfully written book by a well-known professor which uniquely combines theoretical positions with clinical advice.

─────────────────────── ONLINE RESOURCES ───────────────────────

- The British Psychological Society: www.bps.org.uk
- NHS England, Adult Improving Access to Psychological Therapies: www.england.nhs.uk/mental-health/adults/iapt
- Dynamic Interpersonal Therapy (DIT): www.d-i-t.org
- British Psychoanalytic Council: www.bpc.org.uk

REFERENCES

Abbas, A. A., Kisely, S. R., Town, J. M., Leichsenring, F., Driessen, E., De Maat, S., Gerber, A., Dekker, J., Rabung, S., Rusalovska, S., & Crowe E. (2014). Short-term psychodynamic psychotherapies for common mental disorders. *Cochrane Database of Systematic Reviews*, 17. DOI: 10.1002/14651858.CD004687

Abrahams, D. (2017). Dynamic Interpersonal Therapy: Working with perceptions of self and other. *Counselling and Psychotherapy Journal*, 7(3), 8–13.

Allen, J. P., Moore, C., Kuperminc, G., & Bell, K. (1998). Attachment and adolescent psychosocial functioning. *Child Development, 69*(5), 1406–1419.

Barr, N. (2004). *The economics of the welfare state.* Oxford: Oxford University Press.

Bartholomew, K. & Horowitz, L. M. (1991). Attachment styles among young adults: A test of a four-category model. *Journal of Personality and Social Psychology, 61*, 226–244.

Blatt, S. & Homman, E. (1992). Parent–child interaction in the etiology of dependent and self-critical depression. *Clinical Psychology Review, 12*, 47–91.

Bordne, W. (1999). Chapter 1: Pluralism, pragmatism, and the therapeutic endeavor in brief dynamic treatment. *Psychoanalytic Social Work, 6*(3–4), 7–42.

Bowlby, J. (1969/1982). *Attachment and loss: Vol. 1. Attachment.* New York: Basic Books.

Breuer, J. & Freud, S. (1895). *Studies on hysteria.* Standard Edition. London: Hogarth Press.

Burnette, J. L., Davis, D. E., Green, J. D., Worthington, E. L., & Bradfield, E. (2009). Insecure attachment and depressive symptoms: The mediating role of rumination, empathy, and forgiveness. *Personality and Individual Differences, 46*, 276–280.

Care Services Improvement Partnership (CSIP) (2007). *Commissioning a brighter future: Improving access to psychological therapies.* London: CSIP.

Fenichel, O. (1996). *The psychoanalytic theory of neurosis.* New York: W.W. Norton.

Fonagy, P. & Target, M. (1997). Attachment and reflective function: Their role in self-organization. *Development and Psychopathology, 9*, 679–700.

Fonagy, P., Gergely, G., Jurist, G., & Target, M. (2002). *Affect regulation, mentalization and the development of the self.* London: Karnac Books.

Fonagy, P., Steele, H., Moran, G., Steele, M., & Higgitt, A. (1991). The capacity for understanding mental states: The reflective self in parent and child and its significance for security of attachment. *Infant Mental Health Journal, 13*, 200–217.

Freud, S. (1914). 'Remembering,' repeating' and 'working-through' (Further recommendations on the technique of psycho-analysis II). *Standard Edition, Vol. 12*, pp. 145–157.

Freud, S. (1923). *The ego and the id.* Standard Edition, *Vol. 19*, pp. 1–66.

Freud, S. (1937). Analysis terminable and interminable. *International Journal of Psychoanalysis, 18*, 373–405.

Glickauf-Hughes, C. & Wells, M. (1997). *Object relations psychotherapy: An individualized and interactive approach to diagnosis and treatment.* London: Karnac Books.

Gomez, L. (1997). *An introduction to object relations.* London: Free Association Books.

Halewood, A. (2017). Psychodynamic counselling psychology. In D. Murphy (ed.), *Counselling psychology: A textbook for study and practice* (pp. 89–103). Chichester: Wiley & Sons.

Kernberg, O. (1980). *Internal world and external reality: Object relations theory applied.* New York: Aronson.

Lemma, A., Target, M., & Fonagy, P. (2011a). *Brief dynamic interpersonal therapy: A clinician's guide.* Oxford: Oxford University Press.

Lemma, A., Target, M., & Fonagy, P. (2011b). The development of a brief psychodynamic intervention (dynamic interpersonal therapy) and its application to depression: A pilot study. *Psychiatry: Biological and Interpersonal Processes, 74*(1), 41–48.

Mander, G. (2000). *A psychodynamic approach to brief therapy*. London: Sage

Ogden, T. H. (1992). Comments on transference and countertransference in the initial analytic meeting. *Psychoanalytic Enquiry, 12,* 225–247.

Petosz, A. (1999). *Freud, psychoanalysis and symbolism.* Cambridge: Cambridge University Press.

Redit.org.uk (2012). *Randomised Evaluation of Dynamic Interpersonal Therapy* (REDIT). [Online]. Available at: www.redit.org.uk/why.php [accessed 27 September 2017].

Roberts, J., Gotlib, I. H., & Kassel, J. D. (1996). Adult attachment security and symptoms of depression: The mediating role of dysfunctional attitudes and low self-esteem. *Personality and Individual Differences, 70*(2), 310–320.

Roth, A. & Pilling, S. (2007). *Competencies required to deliver effective cognitive and behaviour therapy for people with depression and with anxiety disorders* [online]. London: HMSO, Department of Health. Available at: www.ucl.ac.uk/CORE [accessed 27 September 2017].

Shedler, J. (2010). The efficacy of psychodynamic psychotherapy. *American Psychologist, 65,* 98–109.

Spangler, G. & Zimmermann, P. (1999). Attachment representation and emotion regulation in adolescents: A psychobiological perspective on internal working models. *Attachment and Human Development, 1*(3), 270–290.

Sullivan, H. S. (1953). *The interpersonal theory of psychiatry.* New York: W.W. Norton.

Winnicott, D. W. (1953). Transitional objects and transitional phenomena: A study of the first not-me possession. *International Journal of Psycho-Analysis, 24,* 89–97.

Winnicott, D. W. (1960). The theory of the parent–infant relationship. *The International Journal of Psycho-Analysis, 41,* 585–595.

Wright, D. & Abrahams, D. (2015). An investigation into the effectiveness of dynamic interpersonal therapy (DIT) as a treatment for depression and anxiety in IAPT. *Psychoanalytic Psychotherapy, 29*(2), 160–170.

Wu, C. (2009). The relationship between attachment style and self-concept clarity: The mediation effect of self-esteem. *Personality and Individual Differences, 47*(1), 42–46.

8

COGNITIVE ANALYTIC THERAPY AND PSYCHODYNAMIC INTERPERSONAL THERAPY

CLIVE TURPIN

INTRODUCTION

Cognitive Analytic Therapy (CAT) and Psychodynamic Interpersonal Therapy (PIT) are traditionally offered over a four- to six-month period (16 or 24 sessions), although both modalities have been used for shorter interventions (between one and eight sessions). This chapter will explore both CAT and PIT, considering common themes and differences between the approaches in brief therapy settings, both of which can be adapted for people experiencing a range of psychological difficulties.

CAT and PIT are both relational models of therapy, although differ in terms of techniques and frameworks, despite their psychodynamic roots. For instance, CAT employs a variety of applications and is particularly versatile, whether in very brief or more standard time frames. Like CAT, PIT has also been used in diverse fields.

PRACTICAL GUIDE: CAT

At the heart of CAT is the notion of reciprocal roles and thinking about how someone relates to themselves, to others and how they expect to be related to. For example, a person's relational style will have been shaped through early life parent/carer relation-ships in particular, with key attachment figures providing the framework for how the child thinks, feels and experiences themselves and others in relationships and the wider world. The first part of CAT works towards establishing these patterns, relationships and experiences, which influence actions and behaviours. This rich information contributes to developing a written reformulation in an attempt to share a relational understanding of the difficulties and how past events and relationships have played a part in shaping this. The letter is read out by the therapist and approached as a focus and framework for therapy. CAT uses mapping to track thoughts, feelings, beliefs and actions to increase the client's awareness of the patterns that have become established ways of coping or managing with what are often limited resources. The mapping process evolves with the conversation, from recognition towards revision and developing exits or strategies so that a focus for the work can be identified. Through this process, both explicitly and implicitly, a move towards 'healthier' relational roles is developed.

PRACTICAL GUIDE: PIT

Within PIT, also known as the Conversational Model, the focus is upon the 'here and now' and what is occurring in the room between 'I and we' (therapist and client), where the conversation is developed further using a number of hypotheses. For example, hypoth-eses include: understanding – picking up on feelings and the emotional impact of what is being shared; linking – bringing together what is being experienced in the here and now and how this might link with other experiences that have been shared; and finally, the explanatory hypothesis, which can serve as a mini-formulation. All of these aspects become intrinsic in establishing a joint understanding of the problem. There is a strong focus on feelings and the value in tentatively seeking permission to stay with emotions to see what occurs. Metaphors are actively encouraged, as they often become powerful vehicles to a greater, developed felt sense of something and the resulting deepening con-nection and understanding.

EVIDENCE BASE

When CAT was developed, it was designed to be researchable, and its popularity has translated to a greater proportion of practice-based studies over controlled clinical efficacy trials of evidence-based practice. For a comprehensive review of CAT's practice and evi-dence base, see Calvert and Kellett (2014), which suggests that CAT is effective in routine clinical practice and under clinical trial conditions for a diverse range of difficulties.

The evidence-base for PIT indicates that it is an effective treatment for depression, some somatic disorders, particularly chronic, unexplained pain and irritable bowel syndrome, self-harm and psychosis (for an overview of the treatment and evidence, see Guthrie & Moghavemi, 2013).

Both CAT and PIT have been used in brief forms of therapy (predominantly from two to five sessions), working contextually with teams, promoting greater relational awareness for practitioners and trainees, and in the context of self-harm and general mood and relational difficulties (Aveline, 2001; Barkham, 1989; Carradice, 2004; Cowmeadow, 1994, 1995; Guthrie et al., 2001; Sheard et al., 2000).

Most brief forms of CAT and PIT have in common a focus on formulating a present or dominant issue that led to the client seeking or receiving help. Many brief formats also commence closer to the incident or period of identified need and, as such, the issues can feel more 'live' and accessible in a slightly different way from medium and longer-term therapy or following long waiting periods before starting therapy. Another benefit of brief therapy is that evidence also highlights that the first four to six sessions of therapy is the time of greatest change (Howard et al., 1986).

HOW THE INTERVENTION OPERATES

Very brief CAT and PIT approaches (highlighted in the NICE review of effective interventions for self-harm; National Collaborating Centre for Mental Health, 2004, 2011) require:

- Focus – Collaboration in establishing goals helps to keep the frame in short-term work and identifying any snags to these or the process of change will be an important component to the early conversations.
- Flexibility – Sometimes the focus needs to change and collaboration and negotiation will be key to this.
- Formulation – A good formulation underpins understanding and growing awareness.
- Problem solving and a solution focus – Using formulation and understanding to explore and develop alternative and new ways of relating and managing feelings.

CAT and PIT both employ a progressive nature to moving from gaining a deeper understanding of the problems and the client's feelings, to promoting recognition and exploring alternatives. What can be achieved in the period available differs widely from person to person and is strongly influenced by motivation, timing and readiness for change, as well as the presence or absence of supportive relationships.

The first session of therapy will review the goals and focus already identified for therapy. Further exploration of the relational understanding of the identified difficulty will develop and link the present to the past. This will involve encouraging the expression of emotions and staying with feelings, establishing relational roles, interpersonal patterns and procedures. In such conversations, metaphor can be used to explore and promote deeper understanding and provide a possibly safer metaphorical container to express feelings.

CAT and PIT are active models and very brief therapy requires the therapist to hold a great deal of participation and skill in pacing. Feelings are often avoided or 'cut off from' and PIT's approach of 'staying with' helps to establish some confidence in tolerating and working towards accepting emotions as an alternative to feeling crushed. There might also be a tension here, as 'staying with' feelings can easily become overwhelming and bring the therapist into a powerful, controlling, exposing or humiliating role, promoting a state shift or dissociation due to the intensity of the emotion. Hobson (1985) warns against this and recommends remaining attentive and tentative to the difficult feeling, such as asking permission to stay with a feeling and to see what arises. Working within someone's window of tolerance is essential. In CAT, it is also referred to as the zone of proximal development (ZPD, Vygotsky, 1978). It offers the idea of constructing a 'scaffolding' of what someone can manage and learn and which informs both the pace and depth of the work. Both approaches encourage an attuned approach, particularly in relation to those that might struggle to say 'no'.

Throughout therapy, understanding, linking and explanatory hypotheses are used, extending understanding of the relational pushes and pulls and the limited options available through the person's life, and working with the person's past when accessible. Life charts are a useful tool and can provide an important context for what has informed current patterns of relating and to build ways of managing feelings (see Table 8.1).

Table 8.1 Life chart (reproduced with permission from the Association for Cognitive Analytic Therapy (ACAT))

Year	Age	Difficult or key event	Gave rise to ... or was coped with by...

Instructions: Work out the key events in your life and their consequences, either in promoting resourcefulness and/or leaving unresolved issues.

Active mapping is incorporated to promote the recognition of problematic patterns and challenging thoughts and emotions. In CAT terms, this will include emotional/feeling states and/or reciprocal roles that are most dominant preceding, during and after a distressing event (e.g. self-harm). For instance, emotions can include a sense of rejection or neglect, leading to overwhelming hurt and anger that is turned against the individual, which can then create guilt and criticism of the self and others (see Figure 8.1). The approach of PIT would be to use an explanatory hypothesis to bring these various parts together. Once a dominant pattern that links with the self-harm is formulated, it can be thought about in other aspects of someone's life. Links can be established from other experiences or go back to early life and parental/family/carer relationships, and go some way to show what has informed the current patterns that have been established as a way of coping.

It is valuable and helpful to add a hoped-for place to the map or a way of relating to self and others, which can include positive and encouraging self-to-self statements as well as things that someone is good at and their interests. This can include kind and compassionate stances that are both encouraging and forgiving, acknowledging 'steps towards'.

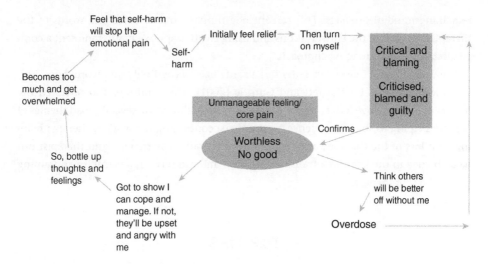

Figure 8.1   An illustration of difficulties presented as a CAT map

Reminders of the negative consequences of certain actions can be useful reflections. Preventative strategies can be explored and employed. 'Letters to myself' are increasingly being used in suicide prevention work, reminding clients of aspects of hope and that difficult moments and distress do pass. Such letters are particularly useful as it can be hard to challenge these thoughts in the moment of overwhelming feelings.

In addition to the map, exit cards (credit card-sized pieces of paper that are portable and quickly accessible) can be used, such as a pause button to promote stepping back and reflecting rather than reacting straightaway. Mobile phones are often the most accessible form of information and resources, and can be used to hold photos of maps and statements or voice file reminders as well as apps and programs.

Endings are approached in much the same way as in other very brief therapies, explicitly stating the number of sessions at assessment and in each session. People who self-harm are recognised to have commonly experienced loss, abandonment and rejection, and therefore the ending can remain prominent through the therapy. The ending of therapy may arrive with some resolution of the problematic issues or a developing new perspective, but it can also be accompanied with possible feelings of anger, disappointment, loss and abandonment. A Goodbye letter highlights the importance of ending, and in being sensitive and attentive tries to introduce a good-enough ending, particularly when endings are so painful.

It is unrealistic to undertake both a CAT reformulation and a Goodbye letter. Therefore, the Goodbye letter begins with a brief written reformulation of the self-harm and the relational aspects of this and how the therapist and patient have worked together, bringing to the letter the depth, difficulties, acknowledgements and progress of therapy. The letter will highlight change, exits or new ways of thinking and aspects that remain work in progress as well as ways of trying to keep the work of therapy in mind, while remaining mindful of snags. This can include thinking of the voice and words of the therapist, imagining the conversations and using creative approaches to represent a compassionate and encouraging approach.

The value of a CAT Goodbye letter has already been recognised and incorporated into PIT research studies by Howlett and Guthrie (2001). These authors also reviewed the impact of PIT Goodbye letters at one-year follow-up, highlighting several broad themes of benefit: helping to share experiences with others; continuing the work of therapy; helping with loss of the therapist and the ending of therapy. The therapy and therapist can be embodied in the letter as a transitional object and can serve as a vessel for containing the memory of therapy.

TOP TIPS

Keep it relational, both interpersonal and intrapersonal.

Attend to feelings.

Try to remain within the window of tolerance to maintain reflection.

Actively work towards change.

CONCLUSION

Very brief therapy has limitations but, as Mann (1973) highlights, it can activate an increased sense of urgency and focus: existentially, time is running out and 'Brevity and depth can be companions, not antagonists' (Aveline, 2001, p. 378). A little therapy at the right time can go a long way. The benefits of a brief and focused reformulation enable a growing awareness and, with it, opportunities to pause, reflect and present an alternative option. By doing so, it can create a new exit to the relational pattern. Focusing on how someone tries to keep the work in mind after therapy is very important and the map acts as a transportable tool, along with the Goodbye letter.

TOP TIP

There are limitations and cautions to be observed in brief therapy. Work within the window of tolerance. In very brief therapy it is important to recognise the complexity of many people's history and the limitations of such brief approaches. It is essential to remain mindful and to actively manage limiting the exploration of traumatic past events. Child sexual abuse is known to be associated with self-harm (Hawton et al., 2002), as is physical abuse (O'Connor et al., 2009), and domestic violence is also a significant risk factor for self-harm (Boyle, Jones, & Lloyd, 2006).

KEY TERMS

Reciprocal roles A role which involves thoughts, subjective experience, feelings, behaviour and the expectation of a reciprocating response from another person. A pair of complementary roles (e.g. loving and caring in relation to loved and secure, or critical and attacking in relation to criticised and crushed) which are most powerfully formed in relationships in childhood, but also later in life. A person may enact either pole of the role and anticipate or elicit (not necessarily consciously) a complementary response.

Exits A way out of a problematic pattern, for instance, a way of relating to others differently, or towards oneself in a more forgiving and compassionate way. They can also involve improving ways of managing difficult thoughts and feelings.

Mapping A CAT tool that tracks the conversation and patterns of relating to self and others on to paper to promote understanding and awareness and to provide a focus for exits and alternatives. Mapping helps in fostering a therapeutic attitude to self and others.

Reformulation Involves establishing therapeutic goals and problematic relational patterns and working towards an understanding of how past relationships and events have informed these. It is anarrative, also conveyed in a letter, offering the client a new and validating understanding of current difficulties, in terms of strategies established to cope with negative experiences in earlier life that currently cause difficulties. It is developed collaboratively and is offered in the form of a letter early in therapy. It will normally identify a focus for therapy.

Hypothesis Used to help promote a dialogue and to work towards a mutual understanding, the hypothesis intimates the importance of getting in touch with and staying with experiences.

Mini-formulation A briefer version of reformulation that has a specific and limited scope, predominantly mapping focused.

FURTHER READING

- Hobson, R. (1985). *Forms of feeling: The heart of psychotherapy.* London: Tavistock Publications.
- Ryle, A. & Kerr, I. (2002). *Introducing cognitive analytic therapy: Principles and practice.* Chichester: John Wiley & Sons.
- Sheard, T., Evans, J., Cash, D., Hicks, J., King, A.., Morgan, N, Nereli, B., Porter, I., Rees, H., Sandford, J., Slinn, R., & Sunder, K. (2000). A CAT-derived one to three session intervention for repeated deliberate self-harm: A description of the model and initial experience of trainee psychiatrists in using it. *British Journal of Medical Psychology, 73,* 179-196.

REFERENCES

Aveline, M. (2001). Very brief dynamic psychotherapy. *Advances in Psychiatric Treatment, 7,* 373–380.

Barkham, M. (1989). Brief prescriptive psychotherapy in two-plus-one sessions: Initial cases from the clinic. *Behavioural Psychotherapy, 17,* 161–175.

Boyle, A., Jones, P., & Lloyd, S. (2006). The association between domestic violence and self-harm in emergency medicine patients. *Emergency Medicine Journal, 23,* 604–607.

Calvert, R., & Kellett, S. (2014). Cognitive analytic therapy: A review of the outcome evidence base for treatment. *Psychology and Psychotherapy: Theory, Research and Practice, 87*(3), 253–277.

Carradice, A. (2004). Applying CAT to guide indirect working. *ACAT Reformulation, 23,* 16–23.

Cowmeadow, P. (1994). Deliberate self-harm and cognitive analytic therapy. *International Journal of Short-Term Psychotherapy, 9,* 135–150.

Cowmeadow, P. (1995). Very brief psychotherapeutic interventions with deliberate self-harmers. In A. Ryle (ed.), *Cognitive analytic therapy: Developments in theory and practice* (Chapter 3, pp. 55–66). Chichester: John Wiley & Sons.

Guthrie, E., et al. (2001). Randomised controlled trial of brief psychological intervention after deliberate self-poisoning. *British Medical Journal, 323,* 135–138.

Guthrie, E. & Moghavemi, A. (2013). Psychodynamic interpersonal therapy: An overview of treatment and evidence. *Psychodynamic Psychiatry, 41*(4), 619–635.

Hawton, K., Rodham, K., Evans, E., et al. (2002). Deliberate self-harm in adolescents: Self-report survey in schools in England. *British Medical Journal, 325,* 1207–1211.

Hobson, R. (1985). *Forms of feeling: The heart of psychotherapy.* London: Tavistock Publications.

Howard, K. I., Kopta, S. M., Krause, M. S., & Orlinsky, D. E. (1986). The dose–effect relationship in psychotherapy. *American Psychologist, 41*(2), 159–164.

Howlett, S. & Guthrie, E. (2001). Use of farewell letters in the context of brief psychodynamic interpersonal therapy with irritable bowel syndrome patients. *British Journal of Psychotherapy, 18*(1), 52–67.

Mann, J. (1973). *Time-limited psychotherapy.* Cambridge, MA: Harvard University Press.

National Collaborating Centre for Mental Health (2004). *Self-harm: The short-term physical and psychological management and secondary prevention of self-harm in primary and secondary care.* NICE Clinical Guideline 16. London: National Institute for Clinical Excellence.

National Collaborating Centre for Mental Health (2011). *Self-harm: Longer-term management.* NICE Clinical Guideline 133. London: National Institute for Clinical Excellence.

O'Connor, R. C., Rasmussen, S., Miles, J., & Hawton, K. (2009). Self-harm in adolescents: Self-report survey in schools in Scotland. *The British Journal of Psychiatry, 194*(1), 68–72.

Sheard, T., Evans, J., Cash, D., Hicks, J., King, A., Morgan, N., Nereli, B., Porter, I., Rees, H., Sandford, J., Slinn, R., & Sunder, K. (2000). A CAT-derived one to three session intervention for repeated deliberate self-harm: A description of the model and initial experience of trainee psychiatrists in using it. *British Journal of Medical Psychology, 73,* 179–196.

Vygotsky, L. S. (1978). La prehistoire du discours ecrit. *Social Science Information, 17*(1), 1–17.

PART II
INTEGRATIVE APPROACHES AND MODALITIES

9

BRIEF USES OF COMPASSIONATE MIND TRAINING

HANNAH WILSON

INTRODUCTION

This chapter will discuss the use of Compassion Focused Therapy (CFT) and Compassionate Mind Training (CMT) as a brief intervention. It will cover the following:

- An overview of CFT and an introduction to its philosophy and aims
- A review of the evidence base for brief CFT
- An exploration of some of the tasks and techniques involved in brief CFT
- A look at the different levels of formulation within CFT and how CFT works in practice through a selection of brief case studies.

CFT is a relatively new model of therapy. It was specifically designed for individuals who experience high levels of shame and self-attack/self-criticism (e.g. Gilbert, 2009). It aims to develop an individual's ability to experience and accept affiliative emotions towards themselves and others; to build the capacity for compassion towards oneself, but also towards others, and to accept compassion from others. Traditional approaches, such as Cognitive Behavioural Therapy, often appeal to an individual's logic and reasoning, but for some this does not help them to *feel* any differently. Paul Gilbert's development of CFT highlighted that this appeared to be linked to the emotional tone with which alternative thoughts were being 'heard'. He noted that for some individuals, they continued to use a bullying or cold tone towards themselves, and posited that our internal dialogues act like social stimuli, which the brain processes in the same way as interactions with others (Gilbert & Proctor, 2006). In response, Gilbert developed a new approach, which aimed to help individuals develop a kinder and warmer tone for themselves.

CFT draws on evolutionary, neuroscience, developmental and social psychology approaches (Gilbert, 2009). It is a transdiagnostic model, which looks to better understand the human experience, rather than specific problems or 'symptoms'. The model defines compassion as 'a sensitivity to suffering in self and others with a commitment to try to alleviate and prevent it' (Gilbert, 2017, p. 11). It looks at the flow of compassion in three different directions: self-to-self, self-to-other and other-to-self.

TOP TIP

Spend some time with someone, exploring what their concept of compassion is. What words or ideas do they associate with compassion? This might include both positive and negative connotations. It can be helpful to think about examples, such as a surgeon, where the compassionate thing to do may be to inflict pain or scars, but only in order to relieve longer-term suffering.

Ultimately, the model seeks to build our experiences of positive affect, particularly those associated with caring for others, and feeling cared for and accepted. The model recognises that our minds are organised and motivated by different goals, and as such seeks to explore and understand the function and motivation behind our different thoughts, feelings and behaviours. As Gilbert and Proctor (2006, p. 359) summarise, the principle behind CFT is that 'some people have not had opportunities to develop their abilities to understand the sources of their distress, be gentle and self-soothing in the context of setbacks and disappointments but are highly ... threat focused and sensitive'.

KEY MESSAGE

For me, one of the most important aspects of delivering a CFT intervention is to ensure a client has understood the basic philosophy of the model:

- We all find ourselves in a life we didn't choose, with a body and brain we didn't choose. We have to figure out how they work, without a manual or a how-to guide. Sometimes our life, body and/or brain do not behave how we would have designed them. But, although this isn't our fault (or of our choosing), we do have a responsibility to try to figure them out, in order to be the best version of ourselves.
- Human life, no matter who you are, involves dealing with tragedy. This includes loss, grief, disappointment, pain, and even death. It's important that we acknowledge

---

> the sadness that this is inevitable; yet also allow it to connect us all as a common factor in being human.
>
> When clients I am working with have truly heard and committed to these ideas, it can be a very powerful moment in therapy.

As part of CFT, there is a series of exercises that are designed to develop an individual's compassionate mind (Compassionate Mind Training, CMT). These are 'specific practices to develop physical and mental competences that facilitate self-grounding, the ability to slow down and take a compassionate focus and orientation to self, to others, help balance different types of emotion and work with life difficulties' (Matos et al., 2017, pp. 3–4). The exercises within CMT can lend themselves to brief interventions, particularly with non-clinical populations or less complex presentations.

EVIDENCE BASE FOR BRIEF CFT/CMT

CFT has been utilised in a number of different mental health settings and has been demonstrated to have a positive impact on self-criticism, shame, depression, anxiety, psychosis and trauma (Gilbert & Proctor, 2006; Judge, Cleghorn, McEwan & Gilbert, 2012; Laithwaite et al., 2009; Lawrence & Lee, 2014). It should be highlighted that there is no specified number of sessions to deliver a CFT intervention. It is generally not described as a brief therapy (not least as for individuals with high levels of shame and self-criticism, there may be additional barriers to overcome within an intervention). Nevertheless, there have been some descriptions of brief CMT interventions within the evidence base. As it is also a relatively new model, the evidence for both CFT and CMT is developing and expanding all the time.

Gilbert and Proctor (2006) delivered a group intervention for 12 weeks, for individuals with complex mental health difficulties. They reported that following the group, participants reported significant reductions in scores of depression, anxiety, self-criticism, shame, inferiority and submissive behaviour. There was also an increase in ratings of self-soothing and self-reassurance. Similarly, Mayhew and Gilbert (2008) conducted a study with individuals who hear voices, where a CMT intervention was delivered on an individual basis over 12 sessions. All participants rated themselves as more self-compassionate after the study. Interestingly, the authors also note that the intervention 'appeared to have a major effect on participants' hostile voices, transforming them into becoming more reassuring, less persecutory and less malevolent' (Mayhew & Gilbert, 2008, p. 133).

Matos et al. (2017) developed a protocol for a two-week brief CMT intervention, which was delivered to 93 individuals from a non-clinical population. The results indicated that the CMT significantly improved participants' experiences of both compassion for themselves and from others. Both CMT and the treatment as usual (TAU) increased compassion for others. In addition, Parry and Malpuls (2017) described an eight-week Compassion in Pain Group, based on CMT principles. This particularly focused on the development of self-compassion. At the end of the group, participants reported a reduction in pain-related anxiety and depression, in addition to an increase in scores of activity engagement, self-kindness and self-compassion.

Personally, I have typically used CFT as a longer intervention, although I have had some opportunity to use its brief forms. I facilitated a one-day CFT workshop for my staff team, which included some experiential exercises. This included asking staff to draw out their own 'three circles' (see Formulation section), doing a soothing rhythm breathing exercise (see Compassionate Exercises section) and also an exercise exploring the function of the self-critic. Many of the staff were new to the model and were not trained therapists. The feedback I received was very positive, and they particularly commented on how it had helped them to think about their own relationship with themselves, and where this might sometimes be rather unkind or uncompassionate. They reflected that it had encouraged them to attend to their own self-care and to be more kind and accepting of themselves.

FORMULATION

The CFT model posits that our brain is made up of at least three types of major emotion-regulation systems. Figure 9.1 shows these systems (adapted from Gilbert et al., 2007), which is sometimes referred to as the 'three circles model'.

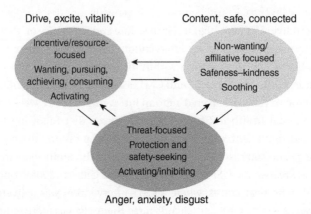

Figure 9.1 Three emotion regulation systems

THREAT SYSTEM

The threat system operates on stress hormones, such as cortisol and adrenaline, and tends to be associated with emotions such as anxiety, fear, anger and disgust. Its function is to detect and respond to any threats and it will activate our fight/flight/freeze/submit response. The threat system is highly sensitive and operates on a 'better safe than sorry' policy; that is, it will treat something as a threat until it is confirmed that it is safe. Often our threat system is associated with rapid automatic reactions, which can occur before we've even fully processed the situation. Each individual's particular automatic reactions are influenced by their learning and experiences, as well as their biology. CFT understands that our 'tricky brains' have evolved to be capable of complex things, such as imagining, planning, predicting and reflecting, while still having an 'old' part of our brain which is driven by basic motives and defensive behaviours. Sometimes these different parts interact in an unhelpful way as we have the ability to become angry, anxious or critical about our thinking patterns, our desires or our past actions.

DRIVE SYSTEM

The drive system is a pleasure-based system associated with feelings of excitement and achievement. It is highly linked to our neural reward pathways and brain chemicals such as dopamine. The drive system helps to activate us to seek out resources and activities that we enjoy. For some people with a diagnosis of depression, this system can be under-activated: they do not experience any drive or motivation to do things or struggle to experience pleasure in things.

SOOTHING SYSTEM

The soothing system brings a sense of contentment and safeness to us and is where we feel soothed and at peace. These feelings are closely linked to our affiliative relationships. When we are young, we require others to soothe and calm our distress. Thus, this system also involves a sense of social connectedness. Physically, the soothing system activates neurochemicals such as oxytocin and endorphins. Gilbert (2009, p. 49) highlights the important distinction between safety seeking and safeness: 'Safety seeking is linked to the threat system and is about preventing or coping with threats. Safeness is a state of mind that enables individuals to be content and at peace with themselves and the world with relaxed attention and the ability to explore.'

Research has suggested that developing the ability to self-soothe and create feelings of self-reassurance can help to regulate a sense of threat (Gilbert & Proctor, 2006). Within CFT, we help somebody to think about how their own three circles or systems can be balanced. Which system is the biggest or which is the one that is predominantly activated? Do they have an understanding of the different things that trigger each system? How does each system interact with the others?

Another aspect of formulating in CFT/CMT is understanding how or why our difficulties have arisen (see Figure 9.2) (for further explanation, see Irons & Beaumont, 2017).

KEY MESSAGE

It is important to note that our systems often interact on multiple levels. So, we may go to work because we enjoy it and get a sense of achievement (i.e. drive), but there can also be an element of knowing we need to go because otherwise we may be fired and lose our home (i.e. threat). We may also engage in something we find soothing, e.g. being with friends, but then begin to worry that we've upset somebody (threat). This is part of understanding how tricky brains can be! We can experience different, even conflicting, emotions about the same thing (e.g. feeling anxious about being angry).

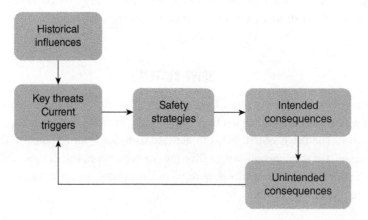

Figure 9.2 Formulation

In brief, the different aspects of formulation are:

Historical influences – we will all have experienced things in our childhood that led us to feel anxious, stressed or upset, which will have activated our threat system. This part of the formulation seeks to understand the different influences on the development of our threat system, be they relationships, experiences at school or specific events.

Key threats/triggers – those early experiences will have left us with particular threats that we are vulnerable to, or with specific fears or concerns. These can be both external fears (concern about how *others* may think, feel or treat us) and internal fears (concerns about thoughts or feelings that arise *inside* us).

Safety strategies – these are the different ways in which your brain helps to keep you safe from the things you find threatening or scary. These may not always seem like the 'right' thing to do, but are usually you doing your best to manage a particular fear or threat. Therefore, what may be labelled as a 'disorder' in one model can be understood as a safety strategy within CFT: 'rather than see these in terms of maladaptive schema or cognitive distortion, they are linked to safety and self-protection' (Gilbert & Proctor, 2006, p. 356).

Intended consequences – these are the intended results, or the function, of the safety strategies you have employed. Sometimes these may be easy to recognise, but sometimes they may take some understanding.

Unintended consequences – these are the side-effects of the safety strategies you have used. It is important to understand that these are *not* things that someone chooses, or wants, to happen – they are unintended. Often, they can be the aspects that lead others to worry or they may mean that people seek additional support or help. I will often highlight to someone that if, when they used their strategy for the very first time, they had known about all of the unintended consequences that would arise, they probably wouldn't have used it. These unintended consequences often end up feeding back into, and strengthening, our threats and triggers, creating a maintenance loop.

This formulation can also be understood in terms of a well-known comic book hero: Bruce Wayne, aka Batman.[1] Bruce's early experiences included witnessing his parents' murder and being unable to do anything to prevent it. This led to key threats and triggers for Bruce of any perceived injustice or unfairness in the world, or of feeling helpless. If he encountered these things, he would tend to feel angry and distressed. Bruce's safety strategy, or way of managing these threats, was to adopt his Batman persona and use his wealth, knowledge and technology to fight crime. The intended consequences of these actions were to make the world safer, but also to feel empowered and effective. The unintended consequences were that Bruce had to hide his real identity, which impacted on his relationships and ability to function in the 'real world'. In turn, he could perceive this as unfair, or outside his control, leading him back into key threats and triggers.

One client I worked with, Matthew, found this way of understanding his difficulties was particularly effective in reducing his shame and self-criticism. He realised that he had not *chosen* to become physically unwell, to distance himself from his family, or to have to leave work. These were unintended consequences of how he had been trying to manage his thoughts and feelings in response to some traumatic experiences, and as such they were not his fault, or 'stupid'. We were able to think about alternative safety strategies that might have similar intended consequences, but with more manageable 'side-effects' that did not impact so negatively on his functioning. Although Matthew still found it difficult to change his behaviour, by using some of the exercises detailed later in this chapter to activate his soothing system and access his compassionate mind, he was able gradually to move towards the version of himself most closely aligned with his values and his hopes.

CFT IN ACTION

CFT is a multi-modal therapy, which incorporates a range of both psychological and body-based interventions. According to Gilbert (2009, pp. 5–6), 'it focuses on attention, reasoning and rumination, behaviour, emotions, motives and imagery'. It draws on approaches used in other models, including 'psychoeducation, Socratic discussion, guided discovery, learning thought and affect monitoring, recognising their source, de-centring,

---

[1] Thank you to Cath Hayes for permission to use this analogy.

acceptance, testing out ideas and behavioural practice' (Gilbert & Proctor, 2006, p. 359). CFT is not a manualised therapy, as the aim is more about changing an individual's tone and motivation in their relationship with both themselves and others, rather than target-ing specific core beliefs or schemas. As Mayhew and Gilbert (2008, p. 116) explain, 'this approach helps people focus on their difficulties in terms of safety behaviours and to become understanding and compassionate to those safety behaviours. ... The therapist helps the person to have empathy for the fear and distress behind safety behaviours and develop tolerance for some of those fears.' There are, however, helpful workbooks for cli-nicians using this model (e.g. Irons & Beaumont, 2017).

Part of a CFT intervention is to help an individual understand their own three systems, including what they are activated, or deactivated, by. The aim of CFT is not to 'get rid of' any of the systems. They each have a vital role to play in our functioning. Instead, we strive to balance the systems, so that each can help to moderate and regulate the others. Too much, or too little, of any system (even soothing) can be problematic. Often clinical interventions will look to develop, or strengthen, the soothing system in order to regulate the threat system in particular. At times, therapeutic interventions may look at develop-ing other systems, for example the drive system for someone who is low in mood and motivation.

CFT uses strategies such as compassionate imagery to generate feelings of warmth and kindness. Individuals gradually develop a sense of a 'Compassionate Other' or 'Compassionate Self', which may take any form (not necessarily human) but possesses the key qualities of wisdom, strength, warmth and non-judgement/acceptance (Gilbert & Proctor, 2006). I have noticed that the majority of my clients find it harder to accept compassion than to give it, and even harder to show it to themselves. However, we can use this to validate that they already know what compassion is, and how to demonstrate it, which is half the work done already. It's just a case of working out how to build their capacity to alter the directional flow of that compassion.

Interventions within CMT relate to the two psychologies of compassion (Gilbert, 2009). The first psychology involves an ability to engage, or connect, with distress, and requires skills and abilities such as empathy, sympathy, sensitivity, distress tolerance, non-judgement and care for wellbeing. Particular strategies, including those from other mod-els, may be employed to build someone's capacity for any of these skills. The second psychology relates to one's ability to alleviate distress, for oneself or for others. This requires skills such as compassionate attention (focusing on things that are helpful or useful), compassionate imagery, compassionate behaviour, compassionate reasoning and thinking, compassionate sensory focusing and compassionate feelings.

In order to activate the soothing system, and to build/access the compassionate mind, CMT employs various different methods, some of which are detailed below. Throughout all of these exercises, participants are encouraged to adopt a warm and friendly facial expression and voice tone (whether internal or not). They are also encouraged to attend to their posture, to ensure they adopt an open and grounded position, which provides a sense of safety and stability (rather than being 'floppy' or tense). Scripts and audio versions of these exercises, and others, can be found in the publications and websites detailed at the end of the chapter.

COMPASSIONATE EXERCISES

SOOTHING RHYTHM BREATHING

This is designed to slow and deepen the breath (Matos et al., 2017), which allows the mind and body to slow down. Research has demonstrated that this can activate the para-sympathetic nervous system and improve heart rate variability, which in turn allows a feeling of being grounded and soothed (e.g. Kirby, Doty, Petrocchi, & Gilbert, 2017; Matos et al., 2017; Porges, 2007).

IMAGERY

Imagery can be a very effective way of activating the soothing system in the context of caring, or affiliative, relationships. Our brains and bodies can respond to imagery as if the thing we are imagining is 'really' happening (e.g. salivating when we think of our favourite meal). CMT employs imagery exercises such as soothing colour, safe place, compassionate other and compassionate self. I have found it is important to ensure clients do not expect themselves to be able to create a vivid, 4D image; usually people create fleeting images, or a sense of an image, and this is typical of a brain (rather than a 'failure').

COMPASSIONATE LETTER WRITING

The client imagines what their compassionate self, or compassionate other, may say in response to a particular difficulty or challenge (Gilbert, 2009). I have seen this be particularly powerful for clients, especially if they are able to read the letters out. It is important that if they do so, they adopt a compassionate voice tone. Often this has been where clients have been really able to connect to a sense that things may not have been their fault, or of their own choosing, and to reflect on their sense of loss around what 'could have been'.

MULTIPLE SELVES

This exercise helps us to understand how different parts of us might conflict, or contradict one another, in terms of their motives, thoughts or behaviours. We invite different parts of us (e.g. angry self, sad self, anxious self) to come forward and explore their thoughts, physical feelings, behaviours, memories and desires. We also consider how those different parts think or feel towards each other and encourage a dialogue between them. The exercise typically concludes by inviting the compassionate self forward, to bring a kind, wise and holistic perspective to the situation and to each of the other parts.

BARRIERS TO COMPASSION

There are a number of potential barriers to compassion, which can impact on our capacity or ability to both receive and give compassion. The Fears of Compassion Scale (Gilbert, McEwan, Matos, & Rivis, 2011) can be a good way to explore this with someone. One particular key barrier can be if an individual experiences kindness as threatening. According to attachment theory (Bowlby, 1980), kindness will activate a client's attachment system, and any associated memories, needs and fears. One client I worked with, Natalie, found any warmth or sympathy from me very difficult to tolerate. We recognised that from her early experiences, she associated receiving care or compassion with threat and/or punishment. Therefore, these fears were triggered by any experiences of kindness or being cared for (Mayhew & Gilbert, 2008). We were able to recognise the irony that for Natalie, she needed soothing in order to feel safe, but soothing itself was currently unsafe.

In my clinical work, I have often found that a particular barrier within CFT has been the strength of an individual's inner critic, that is, their internal voice that criticises them and comments on all the things they've done 'wrong'. It can be helpful to do a functional analysis of someone's critic, to understand what they believe it helps them with. One client I worked with, Stacey, described how she thought her self-critic helped her to strive and achieve things, as it meant that she tried to improve and do better so as to avoid further criticism. However, we realised that when she listened to her critic, Stacey ended up feeling 'rubbish', and like she wanted to 'curl up and hide' (the very opposite of what she thought it helped her with). In contrast, listening to her compassionate voice left her feeling motivated and hopeful.

This was a similar process to my own journey with my self-critic (for further exploration, see Wilson & Joyce, 2017), whom I believed helped me to be the 'best' I could be. Through using compassionate practices for myself, I came to understand and accept my Imperfect Self, and to believe that this was 'good enough'. Although my inner critic is still around at times, I am more able to notice this and to think about which 'mind' allows me to be the best version of me and supports me to reach my goals.

CONCLUSION

Contrary to what some of us might have been led to believe, there is nothing 'easy' or 'simple' about compassion. Behaving, thinking and understanding in a compassionate way takes strength, courage and the ability to connect to and tolerate distress. Helping people to understand that much of what goes on in their brain, and in their body, is not of their design or of their choosing, can be powerful in enabling them to engage in a more compassionate stance towards themselves, instead of one of guilt, shame or self-criticism. Equipping them with skills that allow them to manage the threats and challenges of human life with compassion can have a significant positive impact on their wellbeing, their functioning and their ability to enjoy positive relationships with others and with themselves.

DISCUSSION QUESTIONS
---

1. When you have been compassionate towards someone else, what did you notice about your thoughts, feelings, attention and your body?
2. How might you respond to someone who believes that compassion is 'weak', 'fluffy' or 'self-indulgent'?
3. How do you think the concept of compassion might differ between different groups of people, considering gender identity, cultural background or professional identity?
4. What may be some of the clues that a client you are working with could benefit from a CMT/CFT approach?

FURTHER READING

- Gilbert, P. (2009). *The compassionate mind*. London: Constable & Robinson. This book was the first main published text regarding the Compassionate Mind, and continues to be considered a core text. Dr Paul Gilbert OBE outlines the theory and research regarding the role of kindness and compassion in health and wellbeing.
- Gilbert, P. (2010). *Compassion focused therapy*. New York: Routledge. This book is part of the CBT Distinctive Features Series. It provides a brief but helpful overview of CFT and the different components or skills within it.
- Irons, C., & Beaumont, E. (2017). *The compassionate mind workbook: A step-by-step guide to developing your compassionate self*. London: Robinson. This book provides an updated overview of compassion and practical guidance for clinicians on how to deliver CFT or CMT.

ONLINE RESOURCES

- The Compassionate Mind Foundation: https://compassionatemind.co.uk
- SoundCloud for audio scripts: e.g. https://soundcloud.com/dennis-tirch-phd/soothing-rhythm-breathing
- Compassionate Mind to Overcoming series, all listed at: https://compassionatemind.co.uk/resources/books
- Centre for Clinical Interventions, Building Self-Compassion workbook: www.cci.health.wa.gov.au/resources/infopax.cfm?Info_ID=57

REFERENCES

Bowlby, J. (1980) *Attachment and Loss*. Hogarth P. New York: Basic Books.

Gilbert, P. (2009). Introducing compassion-focused therapy. *Advances in Psychiatric Treatment, 15*, 199–208. DOI: 10.1192/apt.bp.107.005264

Gilbert, P. (2017). Compassion: Definitions and controversies. In P. Gilbert (Ed.), *Compassion: Concepts, research and applications*. Abingdon, Oxon: Routledge.

Gilbert, P., & Proctor, S. (2006). Compassionate mind training for people with high shame and self-criticism: Overview and pilot study of a group therapy approach. *Clinical Psychology & Psychotherapy, 13*, 353–379. DOI: 10.1002/cpp.507

Gilbert, P., Broomhead, C., Irons, C., McEwan, K., Bellew, R., Mills, A., Gale, C., & Knibb, R. (2007). Development of a striving to avoid inferiority scale. *The British Journal of Social Psychology, 46*, 633–648.

Gilbert, P., McEwan, K., Matos, M., & Rivis, A. (2011). Fears of compassion: Development of three self-report measures. *Psychology and Psychotherapy: Theory, Research and Practice, 84*, 239–255. DOI: 10.1348/147608310X526511

Irons, C., & Beaumont, E. (2017). *The compassionate mind workbook: A step-by-step guide to developing your compassionate self*. London: Robinson.

Judge, L., Cleghorn, A., McEwan, K., & Gilbert, P. (2012). An exploration of group-based compassion focused therapy for a heterogeneous range of clients presenting to a community mental health team. *International Journal of Cognitive Therapy, 5*(4), 420–429. DOI: 10.1521/ijct.2012.5.4.420

Kirby, J., Doty, J., Petrocchi, N., & Gilbert, P. (2017). The current and future role of heart rate variability for assessing and training compassion. *Frontiers Public Health, 5*, 40. DOI: 10.3389/fpubh.2017.00040

Laithwaite, H., O'Hanlon, M., Collins, P., Doyle, P., Abraham, L., Porter, S., et al. (2009). Recovery after psychosis (RAP): A compassion focused programme for individuals residing in high security settings. *Behavioural and Cognitive Psychotherapy, 37*, 511–526. DOI: 10.1017/S1352465809990233

Lawrence, V. A., & Lee, D. (2014). An exploration of people's experiences of compassion-focused therapy for trauma, using interpretive phenomenological analysis. *Clinical Psychology & Psychotherapy, 21*(6), 495–507. DOI: 10.1002/cpp.1854

Matos, M., Duarte, C., Duarte, J., Pinto-Gouvela, J., Petrocchi, N., Basran, J., & Gilbert, P. (2017). Psychological and physiological effects of compassionate mind training: A pilot randomised controlled study. *Mindfulness, 8*(6), 1699–1712. DOI: 10.1007/s12671-017-0745-7

Mayhew, S. L., & Gilbert, P. (2008). Compassionate mind training with people who hear malevolent voices: A case series report. *Clinical Psychology and Psychotherapy, 15*, 113–138. DOI: 10.1002/cpp.566

Parry, S., & Malpus, Z. (2017). Reconnecting the mind and body: A pilot study of developing compassion for persistent pain. *Patient Experience Journal, 4*(1), 145–153.

Porges, S. W. (2007). The polyvagal perspective. *Biological Psychology, 74*, 116–143.

Wilson, H., & Joyce, C. (2017). Modelling imperfection and developing the imperfect self: Reflections on the process of applying self-compassion. In S. Parry (Ed.), *Effective self-care and resilience in clinical practice: Dealing with stress, compassion fatigue and burnout*. London: Jessica Kingsley.

10

BRIEF INTERVENTIONS USING ARTISTIC EXPRESSION

LAURA RICHARDSON

INTRODUCTION

This chapter will introduce various approaches to art therapy (also called art psychotherapy), a therapeutic approach using art materials to help with communicating feelings within a therapeutic relationship. Historically, art therapy is rooted in Jungian psychology (see Irene Champernowne, 1968, 1971), psychodynamic psychotherapy and progressive art education. It will demonstrate that art therapy is a 'complex intervention' (National Institute of Health and Clinical Excellence, 2014, p. 218), a client-focused approach, drawn from diverse models and disciplines to suit the strengths and difficulties of the individual and the context of provision. This chapter introduces:

- the role of art in human development
- the benefits of using art in therapy
- art therapy as a distinct practice
- art therapy's theoretical bases
- some theoretical overviews
- some adapted brief art therapy approaches.

ART AND HUMAN DEVELOPMENT

Humans have made art since prehistoric times, and images and symbols have always provided language for experience beyond words. Archaeological finds from ancient South African burial sites show art-related activity from 75–78,000 years ago, and rock art, for example the Coldstream Stone (Figure 10.1), from 9,000 years ago (Marchini, 2017). Depicting three bushmen, it suggests that art has long held ritual and spiritual significance.

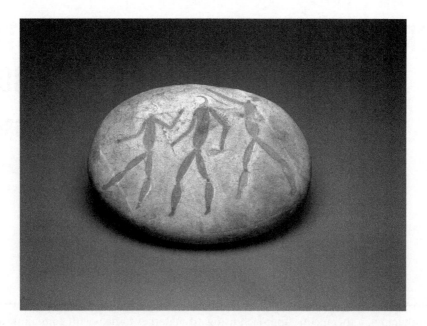

Figure 10.1   The Coldstream Stone (with kind permission of Iziko Museums of South Africa, Cape Town)

Creativity as a feature of human development is thought to have originated when hominids developed into homo sapiens with a forebrain, the pre-frontal cortex. This area governs the executive functions that determine personality and complex behaviour in social contexts (Dingman, 2014). For these reasons, art plays a role in adjustment, resilience, social connection and the expression of community, history, cultural identity and spirituality. Many world cultures also connect arts with health and healing.

ART AND CHILD DEVELOPMENT

The psychoanalyst, Donald Winnicott, defined creativity and compliance as opposite states, contrasting the creative (individual agency in the world) with its opposite extreme, being controlled by others (1971, p. 76). He thought the creative impulse originated in the 'potential space', that is, the reliable and trustworthy environment a 'good enough mother' provides as her baby begins to engage with its world. This process is inextricably involved with a nascent sense of self, and satisfactory experiences encourage the development of imagination and creative use of resources.

THE ROLES OF ART IN THERAPY

The arts are rewarding mediums for psychological therapy, particularly because creativity is relational, forming a bridge between individual and collective experience. Art-making adds spontaneity, increasing the potential for communication through images, symbols, lines, shapes, colours, textures, gestures and marks. It assists by 'externalising' inner experiences and conflicts and working raw materials into an art object can offer experiences of relief and integration (Schaverien, 1990; Leclerc, 2006; Hogan, 2016). Art made in art therapy offers a concrete record, and reviewing it stimulates further discoveries.

SAFEGUARDING

Because aspects of creativity are deep psychological matters, there is a particular need to emphasise 'doing no harm'. For the protection of vulnerable clients (and therapists), specific training in working therapeutically with images and supervision (from a supervisor with specific training and experience) are essential for those intending to use art in their psychological therapy practice. The therapist requires the discernment to respect clients' defences (formed for good reasons) and must appreciate the risks as well as the benefits of encouraging the verbal expression of unconscious material. Malchiodi (2003, p. 13) suggests untrained practitioners risk misinterpreting their clients' communications by unconsciously projecting their own psychological material. Because leaving people more vulnerable at the end of therapy is counter-therapeutic, Springham (1992, pp. 8–16) specified particular care in brief work about opening up areas that would require longer-term psychotherapy to address.

TOP TIP

Creativity involves deep psychological matters. To protect clients, specific training and supervision (from a supervisor trained and experienced in working with imagery) are required from the outset for those using art in their psychological therapy practice.

ART THERAPY

Art therapy developed in the 1940s simultaneously in the United Kingdom and the United States from roots in art practice (Adrian Hill, 1945), psychology and psychoanalysis

(Margaret Naumberg, 1947), and education (Florence Cane, 1951). This intersection ensures a complex and developing international literature. Although the theoretical origins are Western, it is practised in many cultures, and art therapy professional associations exist worldwide promoting professional ethics and encouraging research and development to meet local needs (see Top Tip below).

THEORETICAL BASIS

Prioritising process over product, Case and Dalley (1992, p. 1) framed art therapy as a practice where art materials help with communicating feelings and where no previous art experience is needed. Rather than detached appraisal, there is a shared gaze upon the image where therapist and client allow their vision to 'wander about' in and subjectively 'inhabit' it (Merleau-Ponty, 1964; Maclagan, 2001, p. 36). Where art is appreciatively received, and strengths rather than problems are identified, the therapeutic relationship is a partnership encouraging the overcoming of obstacles. The art therapist is not an interpreter, but instead adopts a 'journeying with' or even a 'following' position with those who might struggle with less collaborative approaches.

━━━━━━━━━━━━━ TOP TIP ━━━━━━━━━━━━━

UK arts therapies professional associations:

- The British Association of Art Therapists: www.baat.org
- The British Association of Music Therapists: www.bamt.org
- The British Association of Dramatherapists: www.badth.org

Worldwide arts therapies professional associations:

- American Art Therapy Association: https://arttherapy.org
- Australia and New Zealand Art Therapy Association: https://anzata.org
- Art Therapy Association of Rio De Janeiro: http://aarj.com.br/site
- Canadian Art Therapy Association: www.catainfo.ca/cata/about-cata
- Caribbean Art Therapy Association: www.facebook.com/CaribbeanArtTherapy Association
- Chilean Art Therapy Association: www.arteterapiachile.cl
- Art Therapy Association of Colombia: www.arteterapiacolombia.org
- French Federation of Art Therapists: www.ffat-federation.org
- German Association of Art Therapists: www.dgkt.de/frameset.htm
- Hong Kong Association of Art Therapists: www.hkaat.com
- Icelandic Art Therapy Association: www.listmedferdisland.com
- Research Educational Association of Art Therapy Iran: https://issuu.com/ artist1366/docs/persian-art-therapy-association
- Irish Association of Creative Arts Therapists: www.iacat.ie
- Israeli Association of Creative and Expressive Therapists: http://yahat.org

---

- Art Therapy Italiana: www.arttherapyit.org/2013/art13_00-home_v15.php
- Korean Art Therapy Association: http://korean-arttherapy.or.kr/index
- Art Therapy Latvia: http://arttherapy.lv
- Arts Therapies Association of The Netherlands: www.vaktherapie.nl/
- Palestine: the Almada Centre for Arts Based Community Development: http://al-mada.ps
- Polish Association of Art Therapists: www.kajros.pl
- Romanian Association of Art Therapists: http://expresive.ro/http://expresive.ro
- Swedish National Association of Art Therapists: www.bildterapi.se/in-english.html
- Art Therapists Association of Singapore: http://atas.org.sg
- The South African Network for Arts Therapies Organisation: http://sanato.co.za
- Taiwanese Art Therapy Association: www.arttherapy.org.tw/arttherapy/tw

Information based on www.arttherapyalliance.org (accessed 29/12/2017) with additions.

THE TRIANGULAR RELATIONSHIP

Case (1990, 2000), Schaverien (1990, 2000), Wood (1990) and Edwards (2004) all described a 'triangular relationship' between therapist, client and artwork (see Figure 10.2). They proposed that one of the active principles of art therapy lies in the integration of communications between these three elements (Edwards, 2004, p. 13). Schaverien's (1992, pp. 79–82) explanations of how transference and countertransference in art therapy are mediated by images through projective identification are seminal in the literature.

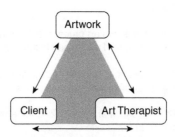

Figure 10.2 Art therapy's triangular relationship (Edwards, 2004, p. 13)

CULTURAL COMPETENCY

Eurocentric understandings of arts, culture and wellbeing do not fit modern practice, making plural, cross-cultural approaches essential. Fanon's concept of 'internalised racism' (1952/1986) remains key for understanding the undermining effects of oppression, as is James's (1998, p. 207) call for psychological therapists to see individuals, families and communities in the context of 'cultural and historical conflicts, confusions and deficits'. Campbell et al. (1999, pp. 15–18) recommend self-awareness around race and culture as vital to effective, non-discriminatory therapy and reflective practice. Recent literature on intercultural art therapy practice assists practitioners to be aware of cultural bias and to adapt art therapy for culturally-specific practice (see Kalmanowitz, Potash, & Chan, 2012; Kerr, 2015).

THEORETICAL FRAMEWORKS

As a flexible approach, art therapy is informed by a range of theoretical paradigms, and some integrative overviews assist with navigation (Wood, 2011).

THE ART THERAPY CONTINUUM

A number of art therapists, including Hogan (2009), Huet and Springham (2010) and Wood (2011), have proposed seeing the work of art therapy within a continuum. In response to changing historical circumstances, Hogan (2009, pp. 29–37) proposed a non-hierarchical list of six strands, known as 'The Art Therapy Continuum', encouraging adaptation rather than adherence to one specific approach (see Figure 10.3).

Art as additional to verbal psychotherapy	Art is a cue for verbal psychotherapy and focused art-making might be introduced if the client seems to be getting stuck.
Analytic art therapy	Psychoanalytically-informed approaches where the artwork is a conduit for the transference relationship between client and therapist.
The group interactive approach	The artwork, the art process, the verbal material and the group dynamics are all addressed in the group.
The individual in the group	The therapist works with each individual and their artwork, without addressing group dynamics.
Art-centred art therapy	The process of art-making and the analysis of the artwork are central to the session.
Art as therapy	The therapist, the art-making and the artwork provide a sense of containment for the client, and verbal interaction is limited.

Figure 10.3 Summary of the 'Art Therapy Continuum'

Huet and Springham (2010) used the metaphor of a bridge spanning long-term and briefer work, public provision and community settings, across which there is movement in both directions. Wood (2011, 2016) advocated therapeutic adaptation in response to changing contexts, with transfers between public, third-sector and private provision enabling greatly different lengths of therapy.

THE MULTI-LAYERED THEORY OF ART THERAPY

Huss (2009, p. 156) used Bronfenbrenner's 'ecological framework' (1979), which depicts human development as movement between social milieus, to explain diverse art therapy models (Figure 10.4).

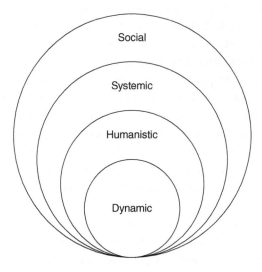

Figure 10.4 Multi-layered theory of art therapy (Huss, 2009, p. 156)

At the centre, the 'dynamic approach' focuses on art about relationships, next are humanistic approaches where art assists with 'taking stock of personal resources' and promoting insight. The penultimate circle concerns systemic approaches focusing on family dynamics and roles, and the outer ring features social models where art is used to explore social contexts.

THE EXPRESSIVE THERAPIES CONTINUUM

Based on the sciences of human development and neurology (later including developing understandings of neuroplasticity), American art therapists Kagin and Lusebrink (1978, pp. 171–180) and Lusebrink, Martinsone and Dzilna-Silova (2013) conceived the 'Expressive Therapies Continuum' (ETC): a stepped model to address early attachment trauma. Clients progress through a series of creative exercises and experiences designed to stimulate different brain-processing areas.

BRIEF AND TIME-LIMITED APPROACHES TO ART THERAPY

In a small profession, once predominantly based in public service but now more widely spread, art therapists are exercised about providing quality approaches which offer the most benefit in a timely manner. The emergence of literature on brief art therapy in the late 1980s coincided with fundamental changes in mental health policy in both the UK and the US. 'Care in the Community', 'Health Service internal markets', 'managed care' and imperatives of austerity have all stimulated briefer approaches to psychological therapy (Richardson, 2006a, p. 11). Currently, art therapists and service users are co-producing consensus clinical guidelines for people with specific difficulties, such as psychosis (Brooker et al., 2007) and borderline personality disorder (Springham et al., 2012).

American psychotherapist Irvin Yalom (1975, 1983), who developed group psychotherapy in psychiatric hospitals, regarded each session as a discreet life span. He recommended a 'here-and-now' focus, highlighting people's positive resources rather than their difficulties. Michelle Wood (1990, pp. 31–35) drew on Yalom when describing 'Art Therapy in One Session' with people with AIDS, suggesting that this helped some with their isolated emotional journey. Springham (1992, p. 10) also turned to Yalom when gearing group art therapy in detoxification care to shorter admissions, advocating full congruence with organisational aims (Springham, 2016, pp. 17–20). Luzzato (1997, pp. 2–10), who also worked in acute care, integrated Hill's (1945) 'open studio model' with Yalom's approach and Mann's 'Brief Dynamic Psychotherapy' (Mann, 1973), to better harmonise with the flow of admissions and discharges.

Further impetus for brief work lies in the widespread adoption of the 'Recovery Model' in mental health care, which Anthony (1993, pp. 4–5) defined as 'a way of living a satisfying, and contributing life even with the limitations caused by illness'. This idea is rooted in the American Christian Twelve-Step Programme from the 1930s, and mental health service user/survivor movements of the 1990s, with borrowings from Chinese, Native American, Canadian and Australian aboriginal and Maori ideas of the community's role in healing the individual. Hope, agency and opportunity are core recovery principles which accord with art therapy's emphasis on prioritising morale and quality of life over diagnosis.

Contemporary practitioners have offered their experience on combining art therapy with a range of brief psychotherapy models (Hughes, 2016), and a summary of some of these adapted approaches follows.

COGNITIVE BEHAVIOURAL ART THERAPY

Solomon (2016, p. 54) noted that 'art psychotherapy and cognitive therapy, in using images, both focus on how behaviour and behavioural change can be observed and measured'. Influenced by Beck (1987) and Ellis (1957), American art therapists Malchiodi and Loth-Rozum (2003) proposed a 6–21 session cognitive-behavioural model of art therapy with a broadly educational approach. They identified the goals as symptom removal and behavioural change, equating images with CBT's charts and worksheets. They found this approach to be effective for addressing self-defeating behaviour through stimulating multiple perspectives, externalising problems and encouraging a sense of self-mastery (Richardson, 2006a, p. 14). Art therapy's mood journals and sketchbooks are also compatible with CBT, and Malchiodi commented in her weblog (2014) on how self-expression improved her clients' engagement with their 'homework' tasks. Combining words and images can also enhance clients' experience of empathy in the therapeutic relationship, helping it to remain 'live' between sessions. Having concrete artwork to review also enhances the ending process.

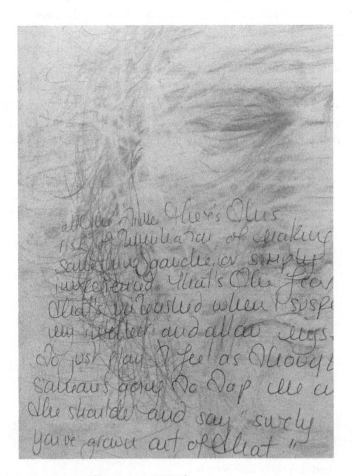

Figure 10.5   'A risky business' (Richardson, 2006b)

Figure 10.5 features a page from the author's art therapy sketchbook, showing the results of 'free drawing' without a plan in mind. An extract of the text reads:

......the fear that's unleashed...... I feel someone's going to tap me on the shoulder and say 'surely you've grown out of that!'

The image explored how perfectionism inhibits play, and shows something of the potential for reflection and exploration along cognitive-behavioural, cognitive analytic, gestalt or psychodynamic lines.

SOLUTION-FOCUSED BRIEF ART THERAPY

Riley (1999; Riley & Malchiodi, 2003) regarded brevity in therapy as especially positive for young people because the implication of temporary difficulty reduces shame. Like art therapy, the Solution-Focused Brief Approach, developed by de Shazer (1985) and Berg (1988), emphasises a partnership approach and focuses on strengths rather than problems. Beginning with the assumption that people who come to therapy are motivated and already resourceful, Riley and Malchiodi (2003) suggested that image-making combined with goal setting, and with parent and child working together, can help any changes to endure. Atkins, a children and young people's art therapist (Atkins, 2016, pp. 119–138), identified imagination at the heart of such tools as the 'miracle question' and 'scaling', explaining that 'art allows imaginings to emerge and be held' (2016, p. 130).

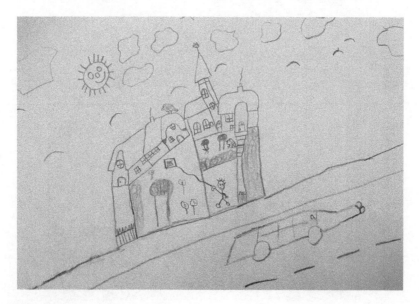

Figure 10.6   'Dad can visit' by Liam (aged 9)

Liam's drawing (in Figure 10.6), made when he was 9 years old, shows him spontaneously using art therapy to imagine in detail how he would like life to be (his story is discussed in full in the Stories from Practice section below).

COGNITIVE ANALYTIC ART THERAPY

Ryle developed Cognitive Analytic Therapy (CAT) to provide time-limited psychotherapy in public health contexts, and this approach shares roots in Object Relations and Jungian Analysis with art therapy. Hughes (2016, p. 49) explained that time-limit and focus encourage engagement and reflection and facilitate empowerment. She synthesised art therapy and CAT to 'better access conscious and unconscious feelings, thoughts and memories', with the CAT elements assisting the release of blocks and awareness of unrealised elements of the self. She memorably explained, 'this integration avoids too much intellectually-based cognitive processing and too much floating in the rich and immeasurable psychic ocean' (Hughes, 2016, pp. 77–78).

PERSON-CENTRED ART THERAPY

Silverstone, a contemporary of Carl Rogers, saw art therapy's ability to access the unconscious as a means of assisting self-reflection. She developed an educational person-centred group approach for the personal and professional development of trainee counsellors. She combined Rogerian empathic listening, non-judgemental acceptance and congruence in the therapist, regarding spontaneous images as 'symbolic aspects of the self in need of recognition' (Silverstone, 1997, pp. 2–3). Contrasting creativity with defensiveness, N. Rogers (Carl Rogers' daughter) valued it for encouraging the individual to 'play' and *go beyond* themselves (Rogers et al., 2012; Hogan, 2016, p. 73). Silverstone proposed four stages in her course: imaging, where 'guided fantasy' encouraged students' imaginations; image-making; making meaning; and working with identified issues (Silverstone, 1997, p. 5).

Identifying affinities between the Rogerian emphasis on authenticity, congruence and empathy and the Confucian philosophy of humaneness, Chang (an art therapist from Hong Kong) described a specific person-centred art therapy approach for Chinese communities. She suggested that the equality inherent in Person-Centred Arts Therapy (PCEAT) can assist with self-direction, 'dignity, satisfaction and creativity' (Chang, 2012, p. 264). Explaining the traditional view that 'emotions disturb the balance of our body–mind–spirit connection' and so also trouble social harmony, she suggested that the arts may offer socially acceptable outlets. Chang (2012) advocated a fusion of traditional arts, philosophies, materials and values with art therapy practice, structuring her approach around a group of Chinese metaphors. These are: the 'five elements of nature' as metaphors for feeling and as departure points for image-making, 'yin yang mandala', where traditional art forms encourage the exploration of internal polarities, and 'knots in the heart', where sculptural knots represent unresolved emotional issues.

MENTALISATION-BASED ART THERAPY

The sense of core emptiness experienced by those with problematic early attachments was described by Thorne (2016, pp. 92–118), an art therapist who explained how this affects people's ability to imagine, reflect and develop a theory of mind (to mentalise). Wood (2016, p. 29) has suggested that although the traditional advice is that those who are 'actively disturbed' should not be offered brief therapy, experience demonstrates that some people with 'disrupted early attachments' may only be able to bear a little therapy at a time. Citing Dryden and Feltham (1992, 1995), whose research indicated a relaxation of such selection criteria, she suggested that, for some, brief art therapy may well be a positive and manageable option.

Bateman and Fonagy (2008) followed consultative NICE Guidelines (2008) when developing their time-limited Mentalisation-Based Therapy (MBT) for use in public mental health services for people diagnosed with borderline personality disorder. Drawing on this, combined with Karterud and Pedersen (2004), Franks and Whittaker (2007) and Springham et al. (2012), Thorne (2016, p. 102) developed a 12-week introductory group, including a series of themed exercises on 'exploration of self and self in relation to other', as one element of a diagnosis-specific programme.

TOP TIP

Drawing on extensive experience of providing art therapy for people with difficult lives, economic circumstances and complex diagnoses, Wood (2016, p. 27) advised: 'There are responsibilities provoked by offering any kind of brief work. These are to ensure there is collaboration with other services, with service user movements, and with community groups: because it is important not to leave people feeling abandoned at the end of time-limited work.'

Thorne (2016, p. 100) noted that art therapy's respect for subjective experience and plural perspectives harmonises with MBT, and in accord with Springham et al. (2012, pp. 8–11), advocated being non-judgemental, 'active in supporting curiosity' about the psychological processes of self and others, and avoiding 'complex or abstract interpretations'. From extensive dialogue with service users, Springham et al. (2012, p. 13) observed that mentalisation is enhanced by the 'repeating oscillation between art making and sharing', finding that the gradual reference between inner and outer worlds seems to help with organising thoughts and feelings.

STORIES FROM PRACTICE

The following vignettes are taken from work in two National Health Service centres and one voluntary sector organisation. Identifying features have been anonymised.

George: Seaside memories

George, a music lover in his 70s who had a learning disability and dementia, lived in an older adult care home for people with complex difficulties. Feeling positive on arrival, he later showed rivalry and aggression towards other male residents. George had been cared for by family members until they passed away, and now he was often lonely, and a heart condition and fading eyesight impeded social activity. Over time, preoccupied with forebodings of death, George was clearly becoming depressed.

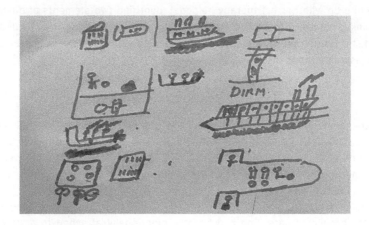

Figure 10.7   'At the Seaside' by George

I invited him to art therapy, where he made this lively drawing recalling a childhood visit to a seaside resort where he remembered its famous tower, boat trips, tennis and a football game (Figure 10.7). George commented 'I can put anything I like on here'.

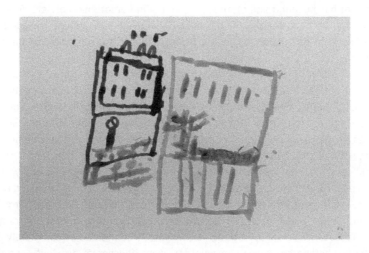

Figure 10.8   'Big House' by George

(Continued)

In a later session, he drew a large house from memory with substantial gardens and allotments (Figure 10.8). He declined to discuss it, but the many windows and chimneys made me wonder whether he had previous care experience, and if this might have affected his orientation to his current situation. George's responses to my weekly invitation were unpredictable, and consent was a recurring theme. Occasionally he shouted and swore saying, 'Can't you see I'm dying?', and sometimes he readily agreed and absorbed himself with pleasure in drawing for an hour. Sadly, following weeks of feeling unwell, George died of a heart attack.

Reflecting on whether art therapy helped, I identified two elements of quality of life. George linked his sense of agency with wellbeing, saying that drawing reminded him that he could still 'do things'. I also gathered that making memories concrete seemed to give him a pleasurable sense of 'flow'.

Jane: The trouble with relating

I met Jane, a keen walker in her late 40s, near the end of her day hospital care. It was her first experience of mental health treatment for her recurring difficulty with severe depression and anxiety which included suicidal thoughts and plans. She lived with her husband, her mother and her two teenage children, whom she was acutely aware would soon depart for university.

My team was keen to prevent a relapse, and requested art therapy as Jane was struggling with the end of care. She had become emotionally attached to a staff member, worrying greatly about how she would manage without his calm, understanding approach. I offered her time-limited art therapy across the transition to less intensive community team support. Because she loved country walking, I asked if there was a place she felt attached to, thinking that a 'sense of place', the landscape and the seasons' slow changes might offer continuity, refuge and a means of self-reflection. Jane responded with line drawings of places she knew and also made insightful diagrammatic drawings showing how she kept her husband and mother 'at bay' behind emotional barriers. She described finding individual counselling at the day hospital 'a revelation', almost 'too good', because it contrasted with her distanced relationships at home, making them seem 'empty' by comparison.

Jane demonstrated, through her drawings of a harbour town, how discharge left her feeling 'shut out', as if left to face the storm alone in a frail boat, and the quay featured these signs: 'Private', 'Trespassers will be prosecuted'. She shared her lifelong sense of isolation, which arose from an uncomfortable maternal attachment, and it seemed that her role as her mother's carer might have re-stimulated uncomfortable childhood feelings of feeling neither attached nor independent.

After 12 sessions Jane went on holiday. On her return, she drew an island with a causeway that appeared and disappeared with the tides (Figure 10.9). She explained that having spent time gazing out at the island, watching its road flooding and re-emerging, noting the refuges for people who missed the tide, she was beginning to feel that relationships need not necessarily be 'all or nothing', either totally connected or completely detached. The metaphor helped her to wonder whether other degrees of proximity and autonomy might be possible.

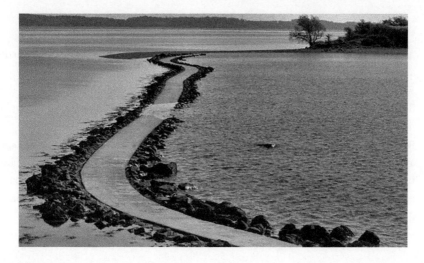

Figure 10.9   Causeway to Rough Island (© Albert Bridge and licensed for reuse under this Creative Commons Licence)

Liam: Location and grief

Nine-year-old Liam, a middle child of three, loved TV adventure programmes and lived in the inner city with his divorced mother and siblings. Following years of domestic abuse, they were helped by a voluntary organisation assisting vulnerable families with children under 5. Contact with Liam's father was sporadic, unplanned and often acrimonious, and this was alarming for the family. As the oldest boy, Liam was torn between protecting his mother and missing his father, becoming withdrawn and uncommunicative as he struggled with his complex grieving process.

Session after session, Liam ignored the art materials, instead diving straight for a Wendy House (which he covered with blankets and cushions), climbing inside and remaining there quietly until the end of the session. I felt challenged about how to respond, but it seemed most important to try to understand his communication. I drew his 'den' and reconstructed it ready for each session, and I occasionally broke the silence with tentative connections: 'I'm hoping you are warm and comfy in there Liam', 'I'm wondering if you are thirsty', but he did not respond. This did not seem like play as I understood it, and I came to see the little house as a refuge or armour against the bewildering adult world. This 'incubation' phase seemed essential to establish therapy as a 'safe-enough place' for Liam to later play and reflect.

During session six something shifted; when I enquired, Liam's hand appeared at the window, and I responded with a cup of juice. For a while, a ritual was established where Liam took the lead. Without pressure, he gradually emerged before the end of the session and spent increasing time investigating the room and its resources. When he drew (see Figure 10.6), Liam conjured a playful scene with himself and his family. A good road enables father to drive over and visit. Notably, father is depicted driving away, and from this I gathered that while Liam wanted contact, he also needed it to be finite and boundaried.

CONCLUSION

- Art-making is intrinsic to human development, making it a therapeutic medium accessing both conscious and unconscious material.
- Art therapy has been developed internationally, within public health services, as a flexible client-focused approach for people with severe and enduring problems with mental health, wellbeing and learning disabilities.
- Rooted in psychodynamic theory, practice is diverse due to practitioners adapting approaches around individual service users and specific service contexts. The literature refers to integrating art therapy with a variety of brief psychotherapy approaches, and positive effects are suggested. Within the profession, efforts are being made to define these approaches for effective research.

DISCUSSION QUESTIONS

1. How do you feel about making and viewing art?
2. In your family, what education and cultural background influences how you feel about it?
3. How might you depict these influences?
4. Imagine a landscape observing all the details. What's the season? What's the weather doing?
5. Might your landscape say anything about how you feel?

KEY TERMS

Arts in health and wellbeing A range of practices where arts and cultural practices support physical and mental health, e.g. arts therapies, community arts, narrative therapies, storytelling, arts as spiritual practice, arts as rites of passage, arts appreciation, healing environments, and shamanic arts practices.

Art therapy/art psychotherapy A psychological therapy where art is made in the context of a therapeutic relationship. Training and registration with a governing body and 'protection of title' apply in many countries.

Arts therapies An umbrella term covering art therapy, music therapy, drama therapy and often including dance and movement therapy.

Borderline personality disorder A mental health diagnosis describing difficulties with emotional regulation, impulsivity, problems with self-image, unstable relationships, feelings of emptiness and self-destructive behaviour (World Health Organisation, 2003).

Client-focused Where the course of therapy follows the client's agenda and the therapeutic relationship is collaborative (as distinct from 'client-centred' therapy, which describes the person-centred methods of Carl Rogers).

Countertransference See *Transference and countertransference*

Creative therapies The range of arts – art, music, drama and performance, dance, poetry, storytelling and play – that can be used therapeutically.

'Do no harm' From the Hippocratic Oath, the Ancient Greek foundation of medical ethics (North, 2002).

Expressive arts therapies The use of art, music, drama, dance/movement, poetry/creative writing, bibliotherapy, play and sand play within the context of formal psychotherapy, counselling, rehabilitation or medicine (Malchiodi, 2014).

Free association A psychoanalytic technique originated by Freud that aims to reveal subconscious influences. The client is encouraged to relax and speak freely without self-censorship.

Good enough mother (see also *Potential space*) 'The good-enough mother … starts off with an almost complete adaptation to her infant's needs, and as time proceeds she adapts less and less completely, gradually, according to the infant's growing ability to deal with her failure' (Winnicott, 1953, p. 93).

Guided imagery This technique from therapeutic mind/body work involves a trained practitioner offering suggestions conducive to mental and physical relaxation.

Mentalisation The capacity to imagine conscious and unconscious mental states in oneself and others; in other words, 'psychological mindedness' (Allen, Fonagy, & Bateman, 2008, p. 3).

Neuroplasticity A neuroscientific concept describing the ability of brain neurons to be pruned or to regenerate on a constant basis, having applications for the study of neuropsychology, rehabilitation and human behavioural change (Shaw & McEachern, 2000, pp. 3–4).

Non-directive approaches Styles of psychological therapy where the therapist does not offer interpretations but encourages the client to elucidate their thoughts, feelings and ideas.

Object Relations School of Psychoanalysis UK psychoanalysts Klein, Fairbairn, Winnicott and Guntrip, and US practitioners Mahler, Kohut and Kernberg saw humans as social beings from the outset, and relationship as the prime motivation of life (Edwards, 2012, p. 54).

Potential space (see also *Good enough mother*) Winnicott meant the interface where the infant can make its first efforts to play and interact with the outside world (Winnicott, 1953, p. 96).

Pre-frontal cortex The area of the brain that houses the executive functions governing personality, sense of self, behaviour and interaction with the world.

The Recovery Model of Mental Health A synthesis of approaches to mental health emphasising empowerment, condition management, social inclusion and an attitude of hope.

Transference and countertransference People sometimes experience feelings in relationship to another which actually emanate from a past attachment relationship. In psychodynamic psychotherapy, this material is worked with for its insight and transformative potential. Countertransference denotes the therapist's affective response to the client, which can (with appropriate training and supervision) enhance insight into the client's difficulties.

––––––––––––––––––––––––––––– FURTHER READING –––––––––––––––––––

- Campbell, J., Liebmann, M., Brooks, F., Jones, J., & Ward, C. (1999) *Art therapy, race and culture.* London: Jessica Kingsley.
- Case, C., & Dalley, T. (1992) *The handbook of art therapy.* London: Routledge.
- Hughes, R. (2016) *Time-limited art psychotherapy: Developments in theory and practice.* London: Routledge.
- Kalmanowitz, D., Potash, J., & Chan, S. (2012) *Art therapy in Asia: To the bone or wrapped in silk.* London: Jessica Kingsley.
- Kerr, C. (Ed.) (2015) *Multicultural family art therapy.* London: Routledge.
- Waller, D., & Gilroy, A. (1992) *Art therapy: A handbook.* Buckingham: Open University Press.
- Wood, C. (2011) *Navigating art therapy: A therapist's companion.* London: Routledge.

REFERENCES

Allen, J., Fonagy, P., & Bateman, A. (2008) *Mentalizing in clinical practice.* Washington, DC: American Psychiatric Publishing.

Anthony, W. (1993) Recovery from mental illness: The guiding vision of the mental health service system in the 1990s. In J. Boardman et al. (Eds.), *Recovery is for all: Hope, agency and opportunity in psychiatry.* London: South London and Maudsley NHS Foundation Trust and South West London and St George's Mental Health NHS Trust, pp. 4–5.

Art Therapy Alliance (n.d.) List of Art Therapy Associations. Available at: www.arttherapy-alliance.org/GlobalArtTherapyResources.html (accessed 29/12/2017).

Atkins, M. (2016) Solution focused art psychotherapy in assessment, treatment and review. In R. Hughes (Ed.) *Time-limited art psychotherapy: Developments in theory and practice.* London: Routledge, pp. 119–138.

Bateman, A. & Fonagy, P. (2008) The development of borderline personality disorder: A mentalizing model. *Journal of Personality Disorders, 22*(1), pp. 4–21.

Beck, A. (1987) *Cognitive therapy of depression.* New York: Guilford Press.

Berg, I. K. (1988) *Clues: Investigating solutions in brief therapy.* New York: Norton.

Bronfenbrenner, U. (1979) *The ecology of human development: Experiments by nature and design.* Cambridge, MA: Harvard University Press. Available at: www.psy.cmu.edu/~siegler/35bronfebrenner94.pdf (accessed 18/12/2017).

Brooker, J., Cullum, M., Gilroy, A., McComb, B., Mahony, J., Ringrose, K., Russell, D., Smart, L., von Zweigbergk, B., & Waldman, J. (2007) *The use of art work in art psychotherapy for people who are prone to psychotic states.* London: Goldsmiths University of London.

Campbell, J., Liebmann, M., Brooks, F., Jones, J., & Ward, C. (1999) *Art therapy, race and culture.* London: Jessica Kingsley.

Cane, F. (1951) *The artist in each of us.* London: Thames and Hudson.

Case, C. (1990) The triangular relationship (3) the image as a mediator. *Inscape: The Journal of the British Association of Art Therapists.* Winter, pp. 20–26.

Case, C. (2000) Our Lady of the Queen: Journeys around the maternal object. In A. Gilory and G. McNeilly (Eds.). *The changing shape of art therapy: New developments in theory and practice.* London: Jessica Kingsley.

Case, C. & Dalley, T. (1992) *The handbook of art therapy.* London: Routledge.

Champernowne, H. I. (1968) Art therapy as an adjunct to psychotherapy. *Inscape: The Journal of the British Association of Art Therapists.* 1.

Champernowne, H. I. (1971) Art and therapy: An uneasy partnership. Available at: www.insiderart.org.uk/userfiles/file/art_and_therapy_an_uneasy_partnership_champer nowne_1971.pdf (accessed 01/03/2018).

Chang, F. (2012) The integrating person-centred expressive arts with Chinese metaphors. In D. Kalmanowitz, J. Potash, & S. Chan (Eds.), *Art therapy in Asia: To the bone or wrapped in silk.* London: Jessica Kingsley.

De Shazer, S. (1985) *Keys to Solutions in brief therapy.* New York: Norton.

Dingman, M. (2014) *Neuroscientifically challenged: Know your brain: Prefrontal cortex.* Available at: www.neuroscientificallychallenged.com/blog/2014/5/16/know-your-brain-prefron- tal-cortex (accessed 19/08/2017).

Dryden, W. and Feltham, C. (1992) *Brief counselling: A practical guide for beginning practitioners.* Buckingham: Open University Press.

Dryden, W. and Feltham, C. (1995) *Developing the practice of counselling.* Developing Counselling Series. London: Sage.

Edwards, D. (2004) *Art therapy.* Creative Therapies in Practice Series. London: Sage.

Ellis, A. (1957) Rational psychotherapy and individual psychology. *Journal of Individual Psychology, 13*, pp. 38–44.

Fanon, F. (1952/1986) *Black skin white masks.* London: Pluto Press.

Franks, M. & Whittaker, R. (2007) The image mentalisation and group art psychotherapy. *International Journal of Art Therapy*, 1.

Hill, A. (1945) *Art versus illness.* London: Allen & Unwin.

Hogan, S. (2009) The art therapy continuum: A useful tool for envisaging the diversity of practice in British art therapy. *International Journal of Art Therapy: Inscape, 14*(1), pp. 29–37.

Hogan, S. (2016) *Art therapy theories: A critical introduction.* London: Routledge.

Huet, V. & Springham, N. (2010) A presentation to the Annual General Meeting of the British Association of Art Therapists. Unpublished.

Hughes, R. (2016) *Time-limited art psychotherapy: Developments in theory and practice.* London: Routledge.

Huss, E. (2009) A coat of many colors: Towards an integrative multi-layered model of art therapy. *The Arts in Psychotherapy, 36*, pp. 154–160. Available at: www.academia. edu/1946129/_A_coat_of_many_colors_Towards_an_integrative_multilayered_model_ of_art_therapy (accessed 18/12/2017).

James, J. (1998) Remembering: Intercultural issues in integrative arts psychotherapy. In D. Dokter (Ed.), *Arts therapists, refugees and migrants reaching across borders.* London: Jessica Kingsley.

Kagin, S. & Lusebrink, V. (1978) The expressive therapies continuum. *Art Psychotherapy*, 5(4), pp. 171–180. Available at: https://doi.org/10.1016/0090-9092(78)90031-5 (accessed 01/01/2018).

Kalmanowitz, D., Potash, J., & Chan, S. (Eds.) (2012) *Art therapy in Asia: To the bone or wrapped in silk*. London: Jessica Kingsley.

Karterud, S. & Pedersen, G. (2004) Short-term day hospital treatment for personality disorder: Benefits of the therapeutic components. *Therapeutic Communities*, 25, pp. 43–54.

Kerr, C. (Ed.) (2015) *Multicultural family art therapy*. London: Routledge.

Leclerc, J. (2006) The unconscious as paradox: Impact on the epistemological stance of the art therapist. *The Arts in Psychotherapy*, 33, pp. 130–134. Available at: http://arttherapycourses.com.au/wp-content/uploads/2016/01/Leclerc-J.-2006.-The-Unconscious-as-Paradox-Impact-on-the-Epistemological-Stance-of-the-Art-Ps.pdf (accessed 17/12/2017).

Lusebrink, V., Martinsone, K., & Dzilna-Silova, I. (2013) The expressive therapies continuum (ETC): Interdisciplinary bases of the ETC. *International Journal of Art Therapy: Inscape*, 18(2), pp. 75–85.

Luzzato, P. (1989) Drinking problems and short-term art therapy: Working with images of withdrawal and clinging. In A. Gilroy & T. Dalley (Eds.), *Pictures at an exhibition*. London: Routledge. pp. 207–219.

Luzzato, P. (1997) Short-term art therapy on the acute psychiatric ward: The open session as a psychodynamic development of the studio-based approach. *Inscape: The Journal of the British Association of Art Therapists*, (2/1), pp. 2–10.

Maclagan, D. (2001) *Psychological aesthetics*. London: Jessica Kingsley.

Malchiodi, C. (2003) *Handbook of art therapy*. New York: Guildford Press.

Malchiodi, C. (2014) *Creative arts therapy and expressive arts therapy*. Available at: www.psychologytoday.com/blog/arts-and-health/201406/creative-arts-therapy-and-expressive-arts-therapy (accessed 01/01/2017).

Malchiodi, C. & Loth-Rozum, A. (2003) Cognitive behavioural approaches. In C. Malchiodi (Ed.), *Handbook of art therapy*. New York: Guildford Press.

Mann, J. (1973) *Time-limited psychotherapy*. Cambridge, MA: Harvard University Press.

Marchini, L. (2017) South Africa: The art of a nation. *Current World Archaeology*, 322. Available at: www.archaeology.co.uk/articles/features/south-africa-the-art-of-a-nation.htm (accessed 18/08/2017).

Merleau-Ponty, M. (1964) *The primacy of perception, and other essays on phenomenological psychology, the philosophy of art, history and politics*. Ed. J. Edie. Evanston, IL: Northwestern University Press.

Naumberg, M. (1947) *Studies of the 'free' expression of behavior problem children as a means of diagnosis and therapy*. New York: Coolidge Foundation.

National Institute of Health and Clinical Excellence (NICE) (2008) *Borderline personality disorder treatment and management: Nice guideline draft for consultation*. London: NICE. Available at www.nice.org.uk/guidance/cg78/documents/nice-guideline-for-consultation2 (accessed 13/10/2018).

National Institute of Health and Clinical Excellence (NICE) (2014) *Psychosis and schizophrenia in adults: The NICE guideline on treatment and management.* Available at: www.nice.org.uk/guidance/cg178/evidence/fullguideline-490503565 (accessed 09/11/2017).

North, M. (2002) *Greek medicine: 'I swear by Apollo Physician': Greek medicine from the gods to Galen.* Available at: www.nlm.nih.gov/hmd/greek/greek_oath.html (accessed 02/03/2018).

Richardson, L. (2006a) An exploration of short-term art psychotherapy in the context of the secondary mental health service. MA in Art Psychotherapy Research, Leeds Metropolitan University. Unpublished dissertation.

Richardson, L. (2006b) Reflective practice image journal. Unpublished personal sketchbook.

Riley, S. (1999) Brief therapy an adolescent invention. *Art Therapy: Journal of the American Art Therapy Association. (16/2)* pp. 83–86.

Riley, S. & Malchiodi, C. (2003) *Integrative approaches to family art therapy.* New York: Magnolia Street Publishers.

Rogers, N. et al. (2012) Person-centred expressive arts therapy: A theoretical encounter. *Person-Centred and Experiential Psychotherapies, 11(1),* pp. 31–57.

Schaverien, J. (1990) Triangular relationship (2): Desire, alchemy and the picture. *Inscape: The Journal of the British Assoociation of Art Therapists.* Winter, pp. 14–19.

Schaverien, J. (1992) *The revealing image: Analytical art psychotherapy in theory and practice.* London: Tavistock Routledge.

Schaverien, J. (2000) The triangular relationship and the aesthetic countertransference in analytical art psychotherapy. In A. Gilroy & G. McNeilly (Eds.) *The changing face of art therapy.* London: Jessica Kingsley. pp. 55–83.

Shaw, C. & McEachern, J. (2000) *Towards a theory of neuroplasticity.* Philadelphia, PA: Psychology Press.

Silverstone, L. (1997) *Art therapy the person-centred way: Art and the development of the person.* London: Jessica Kingsley.

Solomon, G. (2016) Evidence for the use of imagery in time-limited art psychotherapy, emotional change and cognitive restructuring. In R. Hughes (Ed.), *Time-limited art psychotherapy: Developments in theory and practice.* London: Routledge, pp. 153–179.

Springham, N. (1992) Short-term group processes in art therapy for people with substance misuse problems. *Inscape: The Journal of the British Association of Art Therapists.* Spring, pp. 8–16.

Springham, N. (2016) Time-limited art psychotherapy: Theory from practice and teaching. In R. Hughes (Ed.), *Time-limited art psychotherapy: Developments in theory and practice.* London: Routledge.

Springham, N., Dunne, K., Noyse, S., & Swearingen, K. (2012) Art therapy for personality disorder: 2012 UK professional consensus guidelines, development process and outcome. *International Journal of Art Therapy.* Available at: www.researchgate.net/publication/271927490_Art_therapy_for_personality_disorder_2012_UK_professional_consensus_guidelines_development_process_and_outcome (accessed 29/12/2017).

Thorne, D. (2016) Portrait of self and other: Developing a mentalisation focused approach to art therapy within a personality disorder service. In R. Hughes (Ed.) *Time-limited art psychotherapy: Developments in theory and practice*. London: Routledge , pp. 92–118.

Winnicott, D. (1953) Transitional objects and transitional phenomena. *International Journal of Psychoanalysis, 34*, pp. 89–97.

Winnicott, D. (1971) *Playing and reality*. Harmondsworth: Penguin Books.

Wood, C. (1990) The triangular relationship (1): The beginnings and endings of art therapy relationships. *Inscape (Journal of the British Association of Art Therapists)*, Winter, pp. 7–13 .

Wood, C. (2011) *Navigating art therapy: A therapist's companion*. London: Routledge.

Wood, C. (2016) Quick sketches and snapshots for Brief Art Therapy as a time-limited approach. In R. Hughes (Ed.), *Time-limited art psychotherapy: Developments in theory and practice*. London: Routledge. pp. 27–43.

Wood, M. (1990) Art therapy in one session: Working with people with AIDS. *Inscape: The Journal of the British Association of Art Therapists*. Winter, pp. 31–35.

World Health Organisation (2003) *Mental health and behavioural disorders: Disorders of adult personality and behaviour* (F60-F69). Available at: http://apps.who.int/classifica tions/apps/icd/icd10online2003/fr-icd.htm?gf60.htm (accessed 31/12/17).

Yalom, I. (1975) *Theory and practice of group psychotherapy*. New York: Basic Books.

Yalom, I. (1983) *In-patient group psychotherapy* . New York: Basic Books.

11

BRIEF INTERVENTIONS IN HOSPITAL SETTINGS

WILL CURVIS

INTRODUCTION

This chapter will discuss brief interventions within acute hospital settings, focusing on the psychological needs of people with physical health conditions or medical symptoms. It will build on the summaries of different therapeutic models and brief approaches described earlier in the text, discussing integrated, individualised and idiosyncratic approaches to formulation and brief intervention within acute hospital settings, alongside the opportunities and challenges this may present.

A brief note on terminology: it is recognised that the term 'patient' is often avoided in psychological literature due to considerations around the historical problems raised by overly diagnostic and medicalised paradigms of psychological distress. The term is used in this chapter as the people discussed are users of physical health services and are more likely to identify with the term 'patient' than 'client' or 'service user'. I recognise the limitations of the available terms and apologise for any unintended offence this raises. All patient examples are based on real cases with details changed, anonymised and/or amalgamated.

The chapter covers the following issues:

- Physical and psychological wellbeing are interrelated, often in complex ways.
- Coping with a physical health problem can affect mental health, which can complicate condition management. Mood, memory or sleep difficulties can affect

medication adherence and engagement with appointments. Someone with complex or long-term difficulties may find medical treatment challenging due to problems with emotional regulation or the ability to tolerate care. This may lead to frequent hospital admissions, worse health outcomes and poorer quality of life.

- Unmet psychological needs can also drive physical health problems, including medically unexplained symptoms or heightened severity of medical issues.
- Within a formulation-based approach, brief intervention, multidisciplinary working and liaison with external services can support the psychological needs of people with physical health problems.

Although challenges are inherent to working in these environments, significant gains are achievable through the provision of brief psychological intervention in hospital settings.

In this chapter, we will explore:

- Who delivers psychological interventions within a hospital setting?
- The complex relationship between physical and psychological wellbeing
- What approaches are relevant to hospital working?
- What are the aims of brief interventions within hospital settings?
- Challenges inherent to inpatient working
- Evidence-based practice and evaluation of available literature

WHO DELIVERS PSYCHOLOGICAL INTERVENTIONS WITHIN A HOSPITAL SETTING?

I work in an acute hospital as part of a Clinical Health Psychology department (led by the Consultant Lead Clinical Psychologist) within the UK's National Health Service (NHS) offering specialist input into a range of health speciality areas on both an inpatient and outpatient basis. Our main remit across health specialities is to support psychological wellbeing in relation to physical health problems, improve coping and adjustment, and facilitate engagement/collaboration with physical health services. The Accident and Emergency (A&E) Medical Psychology Service aims to reduce frequent attendances through supporting timely assessment, formulation and brief intervention in relation to people who present with physical symptoms driven or exacerbated by psychological factors, including long-term physical health problems, complex pain difficulties and medically unexplained or functional symptoms (e.g. blackouts, seizures, tremors, limb weakness).

THE COMPLEX RELATIONSHIP BETWEEN PHYSICAL AND PSYCHOLOGICAL WELLBEING

Around half of A&E attendances (Blunt, 2014) and 70% of hospital inpatient bed stays (Department of Health, 2012) relate to chronic and long-term physical health problems. People with physical health problems often experience mental health difficulties and common challenges to psychological wellbeing, including depression, anxiety, bereavement and loss, relational difficulties, substance use and trauma. Psychological issues may cause or exacerbate physical health problems. For example, the person may be less able to engage with physical health services or manage their condition effectively, adding to the distress experienced.

Psychological problems can also contribute to the development of 'medically unexplained' symptoms (e.g. recurrent pain, gastro symptoms or functional neurological problems). Physical symptoms underpinned or exacerbated by psychological factors put a significant burden on already overstretched health services, accounting for half of all primary care consultations and a third of those in hospital outpatient clinics (Bass & Sharpe, 2003). Disentangling the psychological factors influencing a person's presentation can be challenging for medical teams, especially within an acute setting where anxiety or stress may be heightened – increasing the severity of physical symptoms seen and confounding the assessment of known medical pathology. This can limit treatment options and prolong hospital attendances/admissions.

Many aspects of managing a long-term health condition may be particularly difficult or triggering for someone with longstanding mental health problems. For example, a person who has experienced abuse may struggle to tolerate physical contact during procedures or examinations. Someone experiencing severe anxiety may find their symptoms so frightening they cannot sit with a doctor and talk calmly and logically about their condition and the treatment or management options available. People with problems in identifying or managing emotions (often resulting from trauma or abuse) may be at higher risk of developing unpleasant physical symptoms through somatisation processes, due to the impact of heightened stress on the body. However, many of the patients we see have begun to experience emotional distress as a direct result of their physical health problems.

The psychological demands of living with pain, difficult physical symptoms or a long-term condition often lead to sleep difficulties, heightened stress, anxiety and low mood. This causes distress and impairs coping and adjustment, while also exacerbating and complicating the symptoms seen and medical intervention. The physical nature of the presentation often means that no referral is made to mental health services.

We cannot separate the social context from these issues; links between low socioeconomic status and poorer health outcomes are well established, with *Fair Society Healthy Lives* (Marmot et al., 2010) highlighting how many key health behaviours known to contribute to the development of chronic diseases follow this social gradient (e.g. smoking, obesity, less exercise, poor diet, treatment adherence). The barriers created by social inequality contribute to long-term conditions and have a 60% higher prevalence rate in the lowest socioeconomic groups (Department of Health, 2012). The NHS faces serious challenges in managing the needs of people with long-term physical health conditions. The importance of a truly biopsychosocial approach to physical healthcare cannot be understated, both in terms of delivering effective and safe patient care, and in providing affordable and sustainable health services for the country.

National policy and healthcare guidance recognise the relationship between physical and psychological health. National Institute for Health and Care Excellence (NICE) guidelines for a range of long-term physical health conditions reference psychological issues, including diabetes (NICE, 2013c), cardiac problems (NICE, 2013a) and stroke (NICE, 2013b). NICE has also published guidance specific to the recognition and management of depression in adults with a chronic physical health problem (NICE, 2009). The *NHS Outcomes Framework 2016/17* (Department of Health, 2016) advocates enhancing quality of life for people with long-term physical conditions (e.g. supporting condition management, improving functional ability and reducing hospital admission). The King's Fund (Naylor et al., 2016) highlights the importance of integrating physical and mental health factors, recommending holistic approaches to supporting people with long-term conditions and medically unexplained symptoms, with integrated models of service delivery facilitating skills transfer between multidisciplinary teams. However, insufficient funding and a lack of service integration are key barriers to achieving the much-lauded politically-driven goal of 'parity of esteem' between physical and mental health services.

WHAT APPROACHES ARE RELEVANT TO HOSPITAL WORKING?

The development of a formulation is a fundamental stage in any psychological intervention process (Johnstone & Dallos, 2013; Sturmey, 2009), regardless of therapeutic orientation. Within this setting, formulation facilitates the recognition of psychological factors, which may relate to the physical symptoms being experienced. A biopsychosocial understanding of the presenting difficulties can facilitate medical treatment (e.g. reducing anxiety around a procedure) or psychologically informed intervention (e.g. coping strategies, joined-up care planning, longer-term psychological therapy, services to support social inclusion, peer support groups).

This approach to clinical practice depends on a flexible approach and the integration of multiple theoretical perspectives and therapeutic methods (e.g. cognitive behavioural therapy, acceptance and commitment therapy, mindfulness-based approaches, solution-focused therapy, motivational interviewing). Given the broad range of presentations seen within these settings, an individualised and idiosyncratic approach to formulation and brief intervention is vital. Often, this will also involve indirect working, including liaising with and supporting other professionals involved, to deliver psychologically informed care.

WHAT ARE THE AIMS OF BRIEF INTERVENTIONS WITHIN HOSPITAL SETTINGS?

While the broad themes of psychological intervention within a medical setting may focus on improving coping and psychological wellbeing, additional considerations are often relevant. For example, a piece of work may aim to support engagement with acute/community services to reduce hospital admission or facilitate discharge. Unless managed carefully, it is easy to be caught between the goals of the individual and the systemic priorities of the staff team. To provide examples in context, we will explore these challenges through a series of case studies.

STORIES FROM PRACTICE

Case Study 1: Working collaboratively to reassure and educate

In acute settings, brief interventions as conversations may focus on simply helping someone to recognise the cognitive, behavioural and emotional factors contributing to their problem. Sarah, a 21-year-old woman, presented to our A&E department with significant chest pain. After medical screening, I joined the doctors to feedback the results of her investigations. We talked about physical symptoms driven by physiological 'fight or flight' responses to anxiety, and the impact of misattribution of physical sensations.

The doctors highlighted the wide range of what symptoms are considered 'normal'. Sarah felt reassured by the explanations offered. We talked about how she could self-refer to local primary care mental health services if she felt she needed further help. We did not see Sarah at A&E again. However, I saw her recently in a local shopping centre. She was keen to tell me that she had noticed some 'twinges' when she felt stressed, but she had remembered what we had discussed with the doctors and felt able to 'wait and see'. She found things to take her mind off the symptoms and noticed that they reduced naturally. Every time she utilised this approach, she became more confident that her 'twinges' were not physiologically dangerous or a sign of an underlying physical condition, thus making them less anxiety-provoking and reducing their frequency and intensity.

Balancing reassurance with explanation

It is important to accompany reassurance with an *explanation* of the symptoms, within a biopsychosocial framework. Trying to challenge the thoughts by telling someone that they are 'fine' can be actively unhelpful and inadvertently leave the person feeling less reassured. A tentative explanation – acknowledging that we might not fully understand the reasons for the symptoms – can help people to tolerate uncertainty and anxiety. A key factor in the success of this brief intervention was the 'normalising' process of talking through Sarah's concern about her symptoms.

Cognitive Behavioural Therapy (CBT) principles were particularly relevant here. Familiarity with disorder-specific theoretical models and CBT-based treatment protocols for a range of presentations is useful, for example, panic (Clark & Salkovskis, 2009), health anxiety (Warwick, 2004), pain (Main & Spanswick, 2000) and generalised anxiety (Wells, 1997). However, a key skill is integrating concepts in a transdisagnostic manner: using these models as starting points to help understand reinforcing factors of complex problems (e.g. safety behaviours, reassurance seeking and hypervigilance to physical symptoms).

TOP TIP

Listening to and normalising a person's thoughts and emotions can be powerful in helping to contain and reassure. Combine this with an understandable and relatable explanation of what is happening (i.e. a biopsychosocial formulation of the problem) to help identify ways forward.

Case Study 2: Surviving the struggle

Intervention in acute hospital settings is often not about 'fixing' the problem. The emotional distress resulting from physical ill health, pain or hospital admission is often understandable and appropriate. It can be unhelpful to pathologise these normal, human responses as psychiatric disorders. Psychiatric medication might not alleviate distress and side-effects may even exacerbate problems. By prescribing medication to address the 'symptoms' of psychological distress, we risk dismissing a person's needs and undermining their confidence in their ability to cope. Psychological approaches are often more appropriate.

John was a 56-year-old man who had been on a medical ward for over a month. In addition to a serious cardiac condition, John had bowel and bladder problems, causing incontinence and significant pain. The medical team was keen to discharge him home but had concerns about his mood and ability to cope. John had declined antidepressant medication.

I asked John how he was doing. He replied: 'Terrible. Just terrible. I don't think I can deal with this.' He told me about the challenges of living with his long-term health condition and the impact it had on his life. Because of his condition, he was unable to get out of the house or see his friends. We talked about his fears around dying – all underpinned by the constant thought that he could not get rid of: 'I can't cope with this.'

How to tolerate the intolerable?

My role in this conversation was to listen, to really hear what John was saying and support him to reflect on what was happening for him. We talked about how, faced with such challenges, it was understandable that he felt this way and acknowledged the losses that he faced. This helped John to feel calmer and more contained: 'I'm not mad then, eh?'.

Drawing on principles of Acceptance and Commitment Therapy (ACT), I began asking John more questions about his values – who he was as a person. Reflecting on the importance of social contact and his identity as a popular, funny and well-liked man, John found it particularly difficult that he had stopped going to see his friends in the local pub. He no longer felt like the man he once was. However, John noted that, despite feeling as bad as he did, he had managed to build good relationships with the nursing staff on the ward. He took real pleasure in making the nursing staff laugh. I reflected that this seemed a good example of how he was able to do things that were still in line with the core values he held.

We talked about the usefulness of taking a mental 'step back': noticing the thoughts and feelings that are happening without becoming overwhelmed by them. We talked about how striving to push away thoughts and difficult feelings can add to the burdens faced; how acknowledging and 'sitting with' these feelings can free up a little 'mental breathing space'. We discussed the 'struggle switch' (Harris, 2009): the idea that we inadvertently amplify physical or emotional pain by struggling against it. I gave John some cognitive diffusion exercises to practise, encouraging him to label his thoughts as being thoughts, e.g. 'I am aware that I am having the thought that I can't cope with this' (Flaxman, Blackledge, & Bond, 2010).

Adjusting through commitment to valued action

A few days later, John described how a burden had lifted. We reflected on how, given the challenges faced, it was understandable he would feel low at times. This realisation had enabled him to stop criticising himself for not coping as well as he thought he should. Noticing just how much time and effort he put into cheering up the nurses looking after him was a turning point. He told me that, as soon as he was able to get out of hospital, he was going to 'face up' to getting back to seeing his friends. Thinking about values had helped him to identify what he wanted to get out of the rest of his life: 'I'm not done just yet'.

Our conversation helped John to realise that he had to adjust to his situation – and that he had some control over this. He had started to notice when he was having 'unproductive' thoughts, enabling him to choose to take a step towards a more valued action. After leaving hospital, John attended a long-term condition psychoeducation group, where he met other people with physical health problems. He did not feel he needed any further support after this. He got back into seeing friends at the pub and, although he acknowledged he could not do everything he once did, he was still able to go and make people laugh.

John passed away about six months later. I look back on our conversations fondly. In a short time, John's mentality shifted from being stuck in a quagmire of self-doubt, self-criticism and fear into one of hope and optimism. I hope our conversation helped to facilitate this process a little.

Using formulation to guide steps forward

By listening to, validating and helping to contextualise John's feelings, we were able to create space for reflection and self-compassion: 'I need to give myself a break here, don't I?' This enabled us to identify ways forward without jumping into problem-solving mode too quickly (which may have been unhelpful). This formulation-based approach avoided describing John's difficulties as simply 'depression' or 'adjustment disorder', which would have pathologised his feelings and ignored the contributing factors. Helping John to recognise that he was experiencing a normal response to difficult circumstances freed him up to think about how he could cope with his situation and adjust to the challenges ahead.

Working in acute health settings requires the practitioner to acknowledge and work from an epistemological position that considers how the thoughts, feelings and behaviours that people experience in relation to their health/symptoms are realistic, normal and understandable. Assumptions or beliefs may not be incorrect or biased. Third-wave approaches such as Acceptance and Commitment Therapy (ACT), Mindfulness-based CBT and Compassion Focused Therapy (CFT) offer useful avenues for supporting psychological flexibility and emotional regulation. Helping people to notice, acknowledge, redirect and respond differently to their negative thoughts/emotions can facilitate thinking about how they can take steps towards valued actions, such as getting out of hospital, facilitating independence or improving quality of life. John coped with the challenges he faced in the best way he knew how: by connecting with people. I hope that, within the context of a book focused on brief interventions, this example highlights how even one conversation can be vital in supporting, understanding and facilitating change.

Case Study 3: Directive approaches within individual and team working

It is important to be clear on the mechanics of an approach. For example, although there is a culturally-driven expectation that 'it is good to talk' after experiencing trauma, NICE guidance for management of post-traumatic stress disorder (NICE, 2005) does not support offering

(Continued)

immediate 'debrief'. Evidence suggests this can be actively harmful, potentially increasing distress and re-traumatising people without offering appropriate grounding and coping strategies. Instead, we focus on promoting a safe and emotionally containing environment around the person.

Kelly was in a serious car accident. She suffered serious injuries and spent some time on the critical care ward, before transfer to the major trauma ward for further care and rehabilitation. Kelly was extremely distressed and anxious. She cried a lot and struggled to engage with physiotherapy. She experienced flashbacks and nightmares, relating to the event and her experiences in critical care when her level of consciousness fluctuated.

Making sense of the experience

Kelly had no desire to talk about the accident itself, yet I did not attempt to push this. We talked about what she was experiencing currently. I outlined some of the normal reactions to trauma that are often seen, mentioning 'fight, flight or freeze' responses, and how flashbacks and nightmares are common as we adjust to and process what happened. We talked about factors affecting confusional states in critical care, including pain, sedation, unusual sleep/wake cycles, unfamiliar environments and irregular staffing. We talked about the positive and functional aspects of strong emotions. We discussed how anxiety following a trauma can be understood as our brain trying to keep us safe from further harm, but that this may then inadvertently lead to heightened tension and pain (making it more difficult to engage in rehabilitation). Acknowledging this, we talked about how we can work through the symptoms and gradually increase movement, avoiding further deterioration and facilitating improved physical and emotional recovery.

By keeping the focus on the here and now, we made sense of the psychological responses Kelly was experiencing. I suggested mindfulness strategies to try, although Kelly found this too difficult. She found that catching up on TV shows on her iPad was a more effective calming strategy and she gradually found it easier to concentrate. With the support of her friends and family, Kelly described feeling 'normal' again after a few days. Kelly felt confident she could adjust to what had happened and was informed how she could access further psychological support if needed.

Balancing directive approaches with collaboration

Making sense of the emotional distress supported Kelly's adjustment and recovery. My role here was not simply to listen. While remaining mindful of power imbalances, I held a guiding and directive position, offering information, education and advice (Rollnick, Miller, & Butler, 2008). A calm and containing response helped identify a collaborative plan. Consequently, we were able to draw on Kelly's own resilience.

A role for mindfulness?

We quickly abandoned mindfulness approaches here. Mindfulness-based approaches have exploded in popularity in recent years, with an increasing amount of research demonstrating their value in supporting pain management, anxiety and coping with health conditions (e.g. Chiesa & Serretti, 2011). Mindfulness approaches can help people reflect on their cognitive and emotional responses. Imagery and cognitive diffusion principles can be useful in disentangling distressing thoughts and shifting mental attention. This can facilitate a less emotionally-driven response to the challenges of being in hospital (e.g. pain, discomfort, nausea, noise, impaired sleep).

However, caution is needed. The focus of many mindfulness-based approaches is not to 'reduce' the intensity of these emotional experiences per se, but to promote a non-judgemental and 'noticing' stance towards thoughts, feelings and physical states. This can be difficult for people to grasp, especially when they are distressed. Mindfulness approaches that focus on physical sensations have been associated with negative outcomes, such as heightened symptom distress (e.g. Reynolds et al., 2017) and increased pain (Lindahl et al., 2017).

I was given *The Ladybird Book of Mindfulness* (Hazeley & Morris, 2015) as a Christmas present. This title, in their series of delightfully ironic and satirical takes on the classic children's books, offers an amusing but all too familiar misunderstanding of mindfulness-based techniques:

> Anna has emptied her mind and is listening to the world around her. She can hear the neighbours arguing, two ambulances, a burglar alarm, a child crying, and the sound of dubstep coming from a Subaru Impreza. She is also concentrating on her own feelings, like her cystitis. (Hazeley & Morris, 2015, p. 14)

Learning to notice and tolerate unpleasant sensations, thoughts and feelings can seem counterintuitive. Checking understanding is fundamental. Interventions must be based on thorough assessment, positive engagement and a cohesive formulation and understanding of the person's needs at that time, facilitated within a collaborative framework.

Engagement with the multidisciplinary team

With Kelly's permission, I spoke with the nursing and therapies teams about how they could best support her (Figure 11.1). Clinical psychologists integrated into multidisciplinary teams often offer training, consultation and advice. As discussed above, giving clear advice or recommendations can be useful. However, the aim should be to work collaboratively with colleagues to reflect on a situation, explore the reasons underlying a presentation and identify steps forward together – creating a supportive environment by drawing on the expertise and experience of everyone involved.

TOP TIP

Achieve good relationships by working in a friendly, collaborative and positive way. Demonstrate the effectiveness of brief psychological work to engage others in supporting patients in a psychologically informed way.

(Continued)

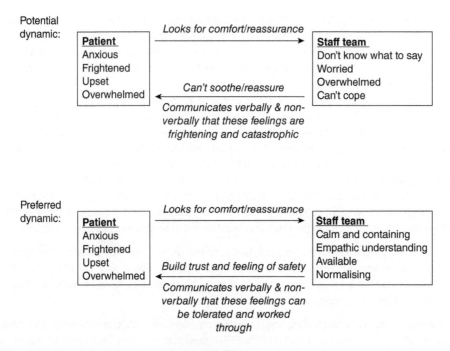

Figure 11.1 Dynamics between a patient and staff team

Case Study 4: Balancing priorities of the patient and the service through collaborative goal setting

Jane, a 40-year-old woman, suffered with increasingly severe back problems. On her fourth ward admission in as many months, neurological examinations and CT/MRI scans suggested mild degeneration of the spine, but no spinal cord impingement. On each previous attendance, Jane received strong pain medication until she could walk with the therapies staff. The medics felt the pain was a flare-up of known pathology, not warranting further admission. When discharge was discussed, Jane became upset, critical of the medical staff and refused further physiotherapy. Situations such as these have the potential to deteriorate into a stand-off, with both patient and staff team becoming increasingly frustrated.

Understanding the role of psychological factors

We began by exploring what Jane's immediate goals were, unpicking what she wanted to get from being in hospital in a collaborative and non-directive way. Quite understandably, Jane wanted her pain to be resolved. She was increasingly frustrated that the problem had been 'ignored'. She worried about the pain constantly. Every day spent in hospital felt like a failure, but when the doctor told her she was 'fit' to go home she felt rejected and abandoned. Fears about not being able to cope with the pain had taken over.

We discussed the role of stress and anxiety in pain, drawing on cognitive behavioural (Main & Spanswick, 2000) and biopsychosocial (Gatchel et al., 2007) models. Considering how psychological and psychosocial factors exacerbate pain, we were able to reflect on why this had become so intense during her inpatient stay. We discussed Gate Control Theory (Melzack & Wall, 1965), which highlights how the brain modulates and regulates pain signals, and how attending to different stimuli affects the degree of pain experienced. This multidimensional conceptualisation of how pain can present at medically unexplained levels provided a meaningful theoretical framework for identifying steps forward. During a session, we captured some of these factors in a diagram to aid Jane's understanding (Figure 11.2).

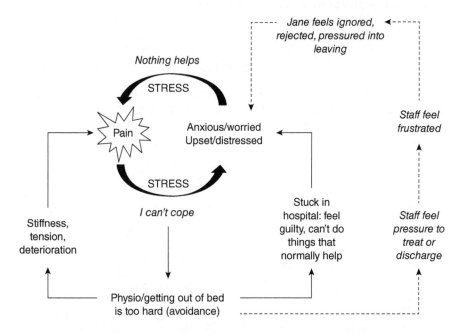

Figure 11.2 Diagrammatic formulation of maintaining factors influencing Jane's back pain

I was upfront with Jane about how I was not providing bedside counselling; we were meeting to discuss her pain, how she was coping with it and what we might do to move the situation forwards. Drawing on Solution-Focused Brief Therapy (de Shazer & Dolan, 2007) and motivational interviewing techniques (Miller & Rollnick, 2002; Rollnick et al., 2008), we discussed what might be different if her pain was more well controlled. What would that allow her to do? What impact would that have on her life?

While there are no quick fixes, I suggested developing a flare-up plan. Working collaboratively with the doctors and physiotherapists, we developed a flexible medication regime (with scope to increase where needed), bed- and chair-based exercise plans (doable even during flare-ups) and mindfulness-based stress-reduction exercises that she could utilise alongside other practical pain management strategies (e.g. ice pack, hot water bottle). The medical team explained what the CT/MRI results showed, acknowledging known physical pathology but reinforcing that the best intervention approach was to stay active. While this did not offer a solution to Jane's immediate goal of getting 'rid' of the pain, it created space for better management of her long-term pain problem. Jane was interested in learning other strategies and we suggested a pain management programme and a chronic pain support group.

Sharing the psychological formulation (Figure 11.2) with the team helped in understanding Jane's presentation and resistance to input. Within a purely medical or diagnostic paradigm, Jane's pain was impossible to fix, as the pathology did not explain the level of pain reported. By disentangling the psychological factors driving or exacerbating pain problems, we were able to take a multi-factorial approach to the pain, creating possibilities for change, while sharing the responsibility for improvement. Understanding the problem from Jane's perspective helped the ward team to make sense of the behaviours they saw, facilitating empathic and supportive responses and reducing their frustration.

TOP TIP

Understand the problem from all of the different perspectives. Drawing on relevant theoretical models and situating the problem within a biopsychosocial framework, collaborate with those involved to negotiate and identify steps forward.

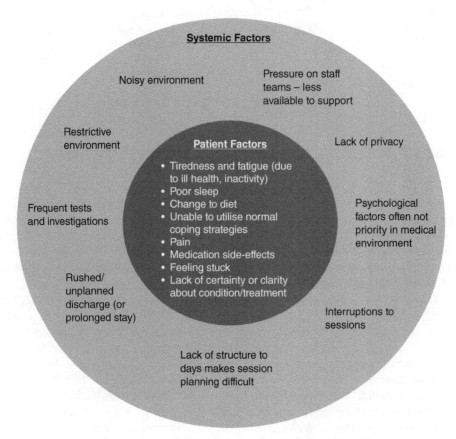

Figure 11.3 Factors that can interfere with psychological work in a hospital setting

OTHER CHALLENGES INHERENT TO INPATIENT WORKING

Figure 11.3 shows other common issues that interfere with working psychologically with patients in a ward setting. Some of these considerations are amenable to change. For example, visiting at a certain time of day can minimise fatigue. If the patient is able, using a quiet room avoids relying on the not-so-soundproof bedside curtain. A harder challenge to overcome is the different philosophies and paradigms that you may encounter when working within medical settings. Understanding distress and emotional responses from a psychological perspective can open up different avenues for intervention beyond psychiatric medication.

EVIDENCE-BASED PRACTICE AND EVALUATION OF AVAILABLE LITERATURE

The breadth of problems seen in acute settings (and the practical challenges involved) means that mechanical, protocol-driven therapies will often be inappropriate. This chapter has focused on integrating theoretical perspectives in an individualised way, driven by idiosyncratic formulation of a person's problems. However, this means psychological interventions can become very different from empirically-based protocols. It becomes harder to quantify outcomes and demonstrate effectiveness through audit and research. In a world dominated by the 'gold standard' of systematic reviews and randomised controlled trials, how do we tailor to the individual patient while being guided by good science?

Clinical psychologists train within a scientist-practitioner paradigm, drawing on available evidence, while utilising skills in critical appraisal to understand the limitations of such research. Within a flexible and integrative approach, they utilise a range of outcome measures, including psychometric tools, goal-based outcomes and the idiosyncratic collection of patient feedback. Consider the use of other service-specific indicators (e.g. a reduction in the number of A&E or GP attendances, ward stay, engagement with care pathways) to help demonstrate effectiveness and value. Psychological professionals working in this context must draw on evidence-based approaches and hold a critical perspective on the strengths and limitations of each. This chapter has discussed various case examples. I would encourage the reader to reflect on the advantages and limitations of the theoretical perspectives and therapeutic approaches used, and on how practice-based evidence might complement evidence-based practice.

CONCLUSION

This chapter has discussed the rationale for the provision of brief psychological approaches within acute healthcare settings, in terms of the psychological needs of people with physical health problems and the impact of psychological factors on medical presentations. A psychologically-informed approach to such presentations can support care and management, with gains achievable for both patients and healthcare services.

This chapter has highlighted the need for integrative and idiosyncratic approaches to care, drawing on psychological theory and underpinned by therapeutic principles of active listening, emotional containment and clinical formulation. Although not intended to be an exhaustive or comprehensive guide, I hope it has served as a useful starting point for thinking about the issues inherent to working in medical settings.

─────────────────────── DISCUSSION QUESTIONS ───────────────────────

1. This chapter has focused on individualised, idiosyncratic and formulation-driven pieces of work with patients with a range of problems. What are the strengths and limitations of this approach to clinical practice?
2. This chapter has presented some practical challenges inherent to acute inpatient work. What others can you think of?
3. What challenges might you face working in a medically-orientated multidisciplinary team? What opportunities could this bring?
4. How can the existing evidence base around brief interventions be adapted for hospital settings?
5. How can teams offer tailored brief interventions in hospital settings?

─────────────────────── FURTHER READING ───────────────────────

-   Fielding, D. & Latchford, G. (1999). Clinical health psychology in general medical settings. In J. Marzillier & J. Hall (Eds.), *What is clinical psychology?* (pp. 259-293). Oxford: Oxford University Press. This chapter offers a useful introduction to the role of clinical health psychologists and is likely be of interest to those seeking to learn more about these kinds of roles within the field.
-   Division of Health Psychology and Faculty of Clinical Health Psychology (2008). *Briefing paper 27: Clinical health psychologists in the NHS.* Leicester: British Psychological Society. This document offers a more detailed overview of the role of clinical health psychologists in the NHS, both in terms of the potential benefits gained through direct psychological intervention and the broader advantages of having psychologists embedded into healthcare teams.
-   National Institute for Health and Care Excellence - Guidance by topic (conditions and diseases). www.nice.org.uk/guidance/conditions-and-diseases. Many of the guidance documents for identification, management and treatment of long-term health conditions explicitly mention psychological issues and outline recommendations for clinical psychology input.
-   Salmon, P. (2000). *Psychology of medicine and surgery: A guide for psychologists, counsellors, nurses and doctors.* Chichester: Wiley. This text offers a broad perspective on psychological issues within healthcare settings, offering insight into the role of stress, appraisals and coping on symptom experience, diagnosis and treatment.
-   The King's Fund - NHS care delivered in a hospital setting. www.kingsfund.org.uk/topics/hospital-care. The King's Fund regularly produce reports and press releases in relation to NHS issues. They have published key papers on A&E performance, NHS waiting times and the interplay between physical and mental health. This website serves as a useful starting point for those wishing to learn more about current issues within the NHS.

- Marmot, M., Goldblatt, P., Allen, J., et al. (2010). *Fair society healthy lives* (The Marmot Review). London: Institute of Health Equality. www.instituteofhealthequity.org/resources-reports/fair-society-healthy-lives-the-marmot-review. This seminal paper outlines the core arguments for the link between social inequalities and health outcomes, offering recommendations for health services and national policy.

REFERENCES

Bass, C. & Sharpe, M. (2003). Medically unexplained symptoms in patients attending medical outpatient clinics. In I. Wilkinson (Ed.), *Oxford textbook of medicine* (4th ed.). Oxford: Oxford University Press.

Blunt, I. (2014). *Focus on A&E attendances*. Nuffield Trust. Available at: www.nuffieldtrust.org.uk/research/focus-on-a-e-attendances (accessed 01/12/2017).

Chiesa, A. & Serretti, A. (2011). Mindfulness-based interventions for chronic pain: A systematic review of the evidence. *Journal of Alternative and Complementary Medicine, 17*(1), 83–93. DOI: 10.1089/acm.2009.0546

Clark, D. & Salkovskis, P. (2009). Panic disorder. In K. Hawton, P. Salkovskis, J. Kirk, & D. Clark (Eds.), *Cognitive behaviour therapy: A practical guide* (2nd ed.). Oxford: Oxford University Press.

de Shazer, S. & Dolan, Y. (2007). *More than miracles: The state of the art of solution-focused brief therapy*. London: Haworth Press.

Department of Health (2012). *Long-term conditions compendium of information*. London: DoH. Available at: www.gov.uk/government/news/third-edition-of-long-term-conditions-compendium-published (accessed 01/12/2017).

Department of Health (2016). *NHS outcomes framework 2016/17*. London: DoH. Available at: www.gov.uk/government/publications/nhs-outcomes-framework-2016-to-2017 (accessed 01/12/2017).

Flaxman, P. E., Blackledge, J. T., & Bond, F. W. (2010). *Acceptance and commitment therapy: Distinctive features*. New York: Taylor & Francis.

Gatchel, R., Peng, Y., Peters, M., Fuchs, P., & Turk, D. (2007). The biopsychosocial approach to chronic pain: Scientific advances and future directions. *Psychological Bulletin, 133*(4), 581–624. DOI: 10.1037/0033-2909.133.4.581

Harris, R. (2009). *ACT made simple*. Oakland, CA: New Harbinger.

Hazeley, J. A. & Morris, J. P. (2015). *The Ladybird book of mindfulness*. Loughborough: Ladybird Books.

Johnstone, L. & Dallos, R. (2013). *Formulation in psychology and psychotherapy*. Hove: Routledge.

Lindahl, J. R., Fisher, N. E., Cooper, D. J., Rosen, R. K., & Willoughby, B. (2017). The varieties of contemplative experience: A mixed-methods study of meditation-related challenges in Western Buddhists. *PLoS ONE, 12*(5), 1–38. DOI: 10.1371/journal.pone.0176239

Main, C. J. & Spanswick, C. C. (2000). *Pain management: An interdisciplinary approach*. Edinburgh: Churchill Livingstone.

Marmot, M., Goldblatt, P., Allen, J., et al. (2010). *Fair society healthy lives* (The Marmot Review). London: Institute of Health Equality. Available at: www.instituteofheal-thequity.org/resources-reports/fair-society-healthy-lives-the-marmot-review (accessed 20/03/2018).

Melzack, R. & Wall, P. D. (1965). Pain mechanisms: A new theory. *Science, 150*(3699), 971–978. DOI: 10.1126/science.150.3699.971

Miller, W. R. & Rollnick, S. (2002). *Motivational interviewing: Preparing people for change* (2nd ed.). London and New York: Guilford Press.

National Institute for Health and Care Excellence (2005). *Post-traumatic stress disorder: Management.* London: NICE. Available at: www.nice.org.uk/guidance/cg26 (accessed 01/12/2017).

National Institute for Health and Care Excellence (NICE) (2009). *Depression in adults with a chronic physical health problem: Recognition and management.* London: NICE. Available at: www.nice.org.uk/guidance/cg91 (accessed 20.03.2018).

National Institute for Health and Care Excellence (2013a). *Myocardial infarction: Cardiac rehabilitation and prevention of further cardiovascular disease.* London: NICE. Available at: www.nice.org.uk/guidance/cg172 (accessed 20.03.2018).

National Institute for Health and Care Excellence (2013b). *Stroke rehabilitation in adults.* London: NICE. Available at: www.nice.org.uk/guidance/cg162 (accessed 20.03.2018).

National Institute for Health and Care Excellence (2013c). *Type 2 diabetes in adults: Management.* London: NICE. Available at: www.nice.org.uk/guidance/ng28 (accessed 20.03.2018).

Naylor, C., Das, P., Ross, S., et al. (2016). *Bringing together physical and mental health.* London: The King's Fund. Available at: www.kingsfund.org.uk/publications/physical-and-mental-health (accessed 01/12/2017).

Reynolds, L. M., Bissett, I. P., Porter, D., & Consedine, N. S. (2017). A brief mindfulness intervention is associated with negative outcomes in a randomised controlled trial among chemotherapy patients. *Mindfulness, 8*(5), 1291–1303. DOI:10.1007/s12671-017-0705-2

Rollnick, S., Miller, W. R., & Butler, C. (2008). *Motivational interviewing in health care: Helping patients change behavior.* New York: Guilford Press.

Sturmey, P. (2009). *Clinical case formulation: Varieties of approaches.* Chichester: Wiley.

Warwick, H. (2004). Treatment of health anxiety. *Psychiatry, 3*(6), 80–83. DOI: 10.1383/psyt.3.6.80.38211

Wells, A. (1997). *Cognitive therapy of anxiety disorders: A practice manual and conceptual guide.* Chichester: Wiley.

12

INTERNET-DELIVERED COGNITIVE BEHAVIOURAL THERAPY

DEREK RICHARDS, ANGEL ENRIQUE ROIG AND JORGE E. PALACIOS

INTRODUCTION

In recent years, computer-based and internet-delivered CBT (iCBT) has become an attractive and evidence-based alternative to face-to-face CBT, and, in some cases, a significantly better option for some individuals. The chapter aims to:

- provide a theoretical background for iCBT and its supporting empirical base
- detail the structure, design and use of iCBT in clinical practice
- illustrate some future developments and use of iCBT in health service provision.

BACKGROUND

In this chapter, our focus is on internet-delivered cognitive-behaviour therapy (iCBT), a descendant of computerised CBT (cCBT). Both approaches are similar in that they deliver evidence-based content. However, they differ in, first, the type of platform needed (a computer with an internet connection versus any computer), second, how service users complete assessments (online versus offline questionnaires), and, third, support is provided for iCBT online or by phone, while in cCBT support can only be provided by phone.

Most computerised and internet-delivered psychological interventions use Cognitive Behaviour Therapy (CBT) treatment protocols, which are especially feasible for being self-applied. Specifically, the didactic format facilitates the operationalisation of therapeutic strategies, and the treatment targets specific behaviours following explicit steps with clearly defined goals (Selmi et al., 1990). Furthermore, Cognitive Behaviour Therapy has the greatest empirical base supporting its efficacy in the treatment of a vast number of psychological conditions (Hollon & Beck, 2016).

The first documented studies of iCBT appeared from the early 2000s and at present hundreds of studies are published about iCBT (Andersson, 2016). There are specific journals (i.e. *Internet Interventions, Journal of Medical Internet Research*) and international associations (i.e. European Society for Research in Internet Interventions) which gather the main leaders and researchers in the field. iCBT has been successfully implemented in various settings and researched for a broad range of psychological difficulties (e.g. depression or anxiety), health conditions (e.g. smoking cessation, stress management) and the psychological distress derived from chronic and somatic conditions (e.g. diabetes, chronic heart disease, chronic pain). What follows is a review of the current empirical evidence supporting iCBT for psychological disorders.

EMPIRICAL RESEARCH SUPPORTING THE USE OF ICBT TREATMENTS

Many studies have examined the efficacy of iCBT for varying degrees of depression, from Subthreshold Depression to Major Depressive Disorder, and in different contexts. The majority of studies concerned individuals with mild to moderate symptoms of depression. Reviews have shown that iCBT for depressive symptoms produces moderate to large post-treatment effect sizes, and they categorise it as a well-established treatment for these conditions, that is, meeting the highest level of criteria for evidence (Richards & Richardson, 2012; Andersson, 2016). Research in internet-delivered cognitive behaviour therapy provided with a supporter continually yields superior outcomes to unsupported delivery formats. A recent review of depression-focused iCBT interventions in primary care demonstrated effectiveness for supported interventions, therefore leading the authors to recommend the use of supported iCBT in primary care (Wells et al., 2018). Similarly, the use of supported iCBT in secondary and community settings is also recommended (Wright et al., in press).

Regarding anxiety disorders, different meta-analyses have shown that iCBT leads to clinically meaningful reductions in anxiety symptoms and increased quality of life (Olthuis et al., 2016). Research in iCBT for anxiety includes Panic Disorder (PD), Social Anxiety Disorder (SAD) and Generalised Anxiety Disorder (GAD). Individual studies and reviews reveal large effect sizes in the reduction of anxiety symptoms compared to controls (Richards, Richardson et al., 2015; Kampmann, Emmelkamp & Morina, 2016; Olthuis et al., 2016). Also, initial research has produced positive outcomes for severe health anxiety and specific phobias (Andersson et al., 2009; Hedman et al., 2011; Andersson et al., 2013; Hedman et al., 2014). Previous DSM-IV anxiety disorders (APA, 2000), including Post-traumatic Stress Disorder (PTSD) and Obsessive Compulsive Disorder (OCD) studies and reviews, have concluded that iCBT interventions are promising (Kuester, Niemeyer, & Knaevelsrud, 2015; Wootton, Andersson, & Rück, 2016). Therefore, iCBT has been proven to be useful in the treatment of a wide array of anxiety disorders.

iCBT research for severe, complicated and enduring presentations includes eating disorders and bipolar disorder. iCBT research outcomes in eating disorder (ED) conditions are promising and superior to waiting list controls, especially for binge eating disorder and recurrent binge eating, leading to reductions in symptoms and improved quality of life (Wilson & Zandberg, 2012; Aardoom et al., 2013). Preliminary evidence supports iCBT interventions for improvements in the psychological and physical domains of quality of life and wellbeing in people with bipolar disorder (Todd, Jones, Hart, & Lobban, 2014). However, the limited evidence prevents firm conclusions about the efficacy of these interventions for such presentations.

Several reports have also indicated positive outcomes for the delivery of internet-delivered interventions to address the behavioural health aspects of chronic and somatic conditions, for example, chronic pain, headache, tinnitus, irritable bowel syndrome and diabetes (van Beugen et al., 2014; Hanlon et al., 2017). iCBT can be introduced as a tailored intervention addressing significant comorbid depression and anxiety in individuals with specific health conditions (van Beugen et al., 2014; Wright et al., 2018). On the other hand, iCBT can be leveraged in disease management, including the provision of disease-specific education, feedback on action plans, medication adherence support and psychological care, to support self-management (Hanlon et al., 2017). To conclude, iCBT interventions have been proven to work for a wide variety of health conditions, addressing psychological difficulties as well as focusing on the behavioural aspects of self-management.

IMPLEMENTING AND RESEARCHING ICBT IN CLINICAL PRACTICE

iCBT delivery can be supported or unsupported. These latter interventions are readily disseminated and mostly targeted at prevention. However, they can suffer from high dropout rates. Furthermore, supported interventions lead to better outcomes and have higher retention rates (Richards & Richardson, 2012; Wells et al., 2018; Wright et al., in press). In this chapter, we put our emphasis on supported interventions, which are delivered by service providers to service users through the means of an online platform, which can be accessed via a computer or mobile device, and which lends itself to direct communication between the service user and the supporter.

Studies indicate that the implementation of iCBT into clinical settings produces moderate to large effect sizes, which are similar to the ones obtained in community samples (Gilbody et al., 2017; Wells et al., 2018). Countries including Sweden, Canada, Norway, Denmark, the UK and Australia have implemented iCBT into routine care

(Titov et al., 2018). In the UK, iCBT is part of the National Health Service (NHS) mental health services (Improving Access to Psychological Therapies, IAPT), whose target is to provide stepped psychological care for people with depression and anxiety disorders. In this case, iCBT is a treatment of choice at step two, that is, for individuals presenting with mild to moderate symptoms of anxiety or depression. iCBT is supported by Psychological Wellbeing Practitioners (PWPs), which are a cohort of graduate psychologists with further training in providing low-intensity interventions. PWPs support service users' progress through the intervention using platform asynchronous or synchronous communication or telephone support. Research in IAPT has demonstrated the effectiveness of cCBT and iCBT in treating symptoms of depression and anxiety (Cavanagh et al., 2006; Richards et al., 2018).

DELIVERING ICBT IN ROUTINE CLINICAL PRACTICE

To illustrate the delivery of iCBT into routine care, we will use the term 'service user' as a category to refer to patients or clients or other users. 'Supporter' encompasses all types of possible supporters: clinicians, PWPs, peer supporters and trained volunteers.

ACCESSING THE ICBT PLATFORM

First, a secure platform is used to deliver the iCBT intervention. This means that all of the data provided by the users is encrypted. To begin, users receive an invitation through email to create an account. Sign-up procedures include creating their username and password and adhere to the latest security and legal standards (e.g. Health Insurance Portability and Accountability Act [HIPPA]; ISO27001 Information and Security Management) and can include dual authentication procedures, similar to the encryption level used in online banking.

Once the service user has logged in, he/she is asked to read the terms and conditions of the platform. This document details the clinical governance standards, including confidentiality and privacy policies, under which the service operates. Information on the supporter and the type of support provided is made available to the user. After the user signs the agreement, he/she is asked to complete some psychological assessment questionnaires. The outcomes of the assessment can be made available to both the service user and the supporter. The user is given access to the platform and the modules of content, including the various interactive tools and the exercises that are offered.

HOW DOES THE ICBT PLATFORM WORK?

To explain the mechanisms of an iCBT platform, as well as its essential features, we are going to focus on the platform we are most familiar with, designed by SilverCloud Health. The platform and content, tools and exercises are continually reviewed by the developers so that they are engaging, effective and informed with the most up-to-date thinking and technology. The platform is composed of four main sections: *homepage, content, tools* and *supporter*.

HOMEPAGE

The user has their secure homepage, and they can decide the content they want to appear on it, generating a sense of ownership. The homepage provides a point of navigation and departure for the service user in navigating appropriately through the CBT content and tools. The homepage also houses the supporter review, the journal and a find help option if they are experiencing a crisis. It is designed using features familiar to social media sites.

CONTENT OF THE PROGRAMMES

The theoretical rationale and treatment focus of an iCBT programme is the same as in a face-to-face treatment, with one difference: the mode of therapy delivery. Face-to-face CBT is mostly verbal; iCBT content relies mainly on text, albeit core CBT concepts and content are presented in many other forms, including videos, animations, slideshows, interactive tools and exercises.

Usually, a programme starts with a brief introductory module explaining how the platform works, the content modules and how to use the tools – an overview that will allow the service user to feel confident in navigating the intervention successfully. The process is similar to what happens in face-to-face therapy, where there is an explanation of the treatment, and the logistics of the work are discussed, such as time of sessions, expected etiquette, explaining the CBT model, the homework demands, and establishing expectations and goals.

iCBT comprises various content modules. The number of modules can vary, depending on the condition treated, but they always start with a psychoeducation module about the disorder or the health state and finish with a relapse prevention module. The modules replicate the content from manualised CBT treatments, either disorder-specific or transdiagnostic. Techniques such as cognitive restructuring and behavioural experiments are included in all of the programmes but tailored for each particular condition. The modules follow a familiar layout to help service users' navigation and familiarity. The core treatment concepts and learnings from CBT are communicated to the service user through a variety of means, including informational content, quizzes, slideshows and videos. Interactive activities help service users understand CBT, for instance, constructing a visual representation of their thoughts, feelings and behaviours cycle. Homework tasks and downloadable files with content summaries are incorporated. The primary goal of all of these elements and interactive activities is to promote engagement with the platform, and also to facilitate the understanding and application of the content and skills.

Indeed, writing content and designing the experience in iCBT is a challenge, and is an area of growing importance. iCBT developers typically include technical content writers, user experience experts, clinicians and designers who create the content for internet-delivered interventions. It is also common to provide personal stories, in the form of video or text, which help service users to feel that they are not the only ones that are having some troubles. Service users are encouraged to follow one module per week, which can take up to 50 minutes to complete. Between sessions, the user is invited to put into practice the learnings of the module, usually through weekly homework tasks. In service-based settings where iCBT is being delivered, deadlines for completing the programme are put in place for the service user. Clear deadlines increase the commitment of the user to the programme and reduce the likelihood of dropout (Andersson, 2014).

INTERACTIVE TOOLS AND EXERCISES

The iCBT platform's technological capabilities can be used to support fully the efficient delivery of the evidence-based content that has been proved to work in the face-to-face context. Developers of iCBT platforms create interactive activities that encapsulate the core concepts and skills of CBT. To this end, a broad range of interactive tools and exercises are available to enhance engagement, promote learning of the cognitive and behavioural skills and strategies and maintain the user's engagement to increase the potential for a successful outcome from treatment. For example, service users can monitor their mood and lifestyle through interactive apps, or engage in pleasurable activity scheduling, which integrates with calendar functions and facilitates the pre- and post-assessment of behavioural activation schedules. iCBT platforms can also facilitate the administration of psychological questionnaires, improving data collection and even the organisation of such data for research purposes.

THE ROLE OF THE SUPPORTER

The meta-analytic evidence to date strongly supports the benefits of guided iCBT interventions for a range of mental health disorders (Richards & Richardson, 2012; Richards, Richardson et al., 2015; Olthuis et al., 2016; Wright et al., in press; Wells et al., 2018). Guided iCBT, either by a technician or a clinician, produces larger effect sizes and higher retention rates than internet interventions without human support (Johansson & Andersson, 2012; Richards & Richardson, 2012; Wells et al., 2018; Wright et al., in press). Regarding the kind of human support, evidence suggests that both technical and clinical support lead to similar results. Therefore, different types of practitioner can provide support if they get adequate training, which is pertinent to dissemination (Titov et al., 2010). iCBT trials, using support from professionals and para-professionals and even trained volunteers, have demonstrated large effects (Richards, Timulak et al., 2015; Gilbody et al., 2017; Karyotaki et al., 2017). These similar results are likely because the role of the supporter is to encourage users to continue using the platform, answering technical questions and providing feedback on homework assignments (Andersson, 2014). In other words, the treatment is the internet intervention, and the support is targeted to encourage service user adherence.

Support for service users in iCBT is scheduled, and supporters can communicate to service users in real time, through telephone or video conference, but mostly support is provided in written feedback through the internet platform. Asynchronous communication allows the supporter to reflect on the feedback they provide to service users. Support time usually takes from 5 to 15 minutes per week, which enables the provision of support to many service users at the same time.

EVALUATION – STRENGTHS AND CURRENT LIMITATIONS OF iCBT

iCBT affords service users as much time as is required to understand the content entirely. Service users have access to their archive of work for a more extended period to re-visit and re-engage with the content and skills. For service providers, maintaining fidelity to the CBT treatment protocol is retained in the standardised delivery of iCBT.

iCBT increases access to services for users who cannot attend face-to-face therapy because of geographical location, physical mobility issues or stigma in accessing treatment. Service providers are better enabled to deliver services to regions and individuals who may not otherwise receive these services.

The flexibility of iCBT is apparent, and service users can fit the time spent online around their schedule, which is important for those with demanding work schedules or other commitments that can be difficult to 'sacrifice' in favour of face-to-face services. This flexibility is also true for the service providers, and supporters can fit the feedback sessions into their working week as they see fit.

Finally, the cost reduction of iCBT versus face-to-face therapy is logical. iCBT realises greater throughput than face-to-face therapy. Healthcare services are beginning to leverage this compelling advantage. It is also true that iCBT is a relatively new field, and thus some limitations exist that merit further study. For instance, poor adherence has plagued the institution of iCBT in regular clinical practice, although it is also true that recent technological developments that focus on the user experience, specifically engagement, are helping to turn this trend towards the positive. It is also the case that some aspects of therapy, such as gentle encouragement to move into exposure or activation, are not possible. But with careful scaffolding and user design features, these can hopefully be overcome. Lastly, there may be less control over service users' utilisation of information (where they may only read and not complete assignments), but this is not necessarily just true of iCBT.

FUTURE DIRECTIONS

As a priority, the dissemination and integration of iCBT on a large scale into clinical practice is still outstanding. Outside innovative services in the UK, Australia and Sweden, for instance, there is much work to be done in achieving a state where iCBT forms an integral part of service user care pathways. Successful integration of iCBT applies to both adult and child and adolescent mental health services. Integrating iCBT in addressing behavioural components in the management of long-term conditions is also important. A significant step to progress is to establish the art of a successful implementation science to achieve large-scale dissemination.

Typically, iCBT has been employed in the service of mild to moderate symptom severity. Some work has examined the utility of iCBT in the service of more severe anxiety and depression symptoms, and the maintenance of remission with iCBT is an area for future research to consider.

iCBT brings the possibility for the globalisation of evidence-based psychological treatments. There is much work to be done in culturally adapting evidence-based treatments for use in various countries and populations, and not just concerning language translation. This is a significant challenge, but work that has already culturally adapted psychotherapy for face-to-face therapy can be used as a starting point for effectively adapting iCBT interventions (Salamanca et al., 2018).

Finally, technological developments may include the potential to use artificial intelligence and ecological momentary assessment. These may lead us to develop more responsive solutions that can more accurately meet service user needs at the individual level, thereby cultivating engagement and successful outcomes for service users (Pasarelu, Andersson, Bergman Nordgren, & Dobrean, 2017).

STORIES FROM PRACTICE

iCBT in IAPT Services

Shivani, aged 37, lived in the UK and worked part-time as a teaching assistant until two years ago when her elderly mother fell and needed round-the-clock care. Shivani gave up her job and became her mother's full-time carer – in addition to looking after her two children. Slowly but surely, Shivani grew more tired, irritable and started having sleep problems. She developed the belief that her life was worthless as she felt that she was a slave to her duties. She felt she would never return to the complete life she knew previously. On a visit to her GP, she completed the Patient Health Questionnaire (PHQ-9) and the GP referred her to Step 2 of her local IAPT service, for the treatment of moderate depression. The service offered Shivani a choice of group therapy or a supported iCBT programme.

Shivani opted for the iCBT as she felt it would be too hard to commute to attend face-to-face appointments. Almost immediately, Shivani was comforted through completing a short online quiz that helped her to understand how common depressive symptoms are in the world. Her comfort only increased as she read one of the personal stories of a woman called Laura, who was also a full-time carer. The behavioural activation module helped her to get back on track and re-engage with her usual activities. The interactive exercises helped her to schedule new activities and she could rate these pre- and post-treatment. What was particularly useful was that she received feedback regularly from her clinical supporter. The feedback focused on empowering Shivani to maintain her activities, which were eventually responsible for reintroducing greater balance into her life and bringing her joy. Challenging some negative thoughts also helped to balance the burden of being a carer and to reformulate her belief that her life was worthless.

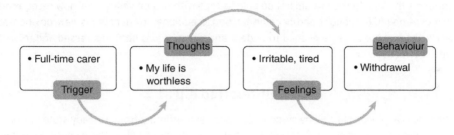

Figure 12.1 Thoughts, feelings and behaviour cycle for Shivani

Table 12.1 Thoughts, feelings and behaviour (TFB) cycle for Shivani

	CBT Core Concepts & Processes		
	Understanding CBT model	**Behavioural activation processes**	**Cognitive processes**
iCBT platform provision of CBT using interactive tools and exercises	**Slideshow on CBT model**	Initial focus on BA through the **Interactive exercise** to schedule, engage and assess pleasurable activities	**Slideshow** of typical negative automatic thoughts (NATs)
	Personal stories in **video** and text of other people's journey and the application of CBT for successful outcomes		**Interactive tool** to create personal TFB cycles and identify associated NATS which are being challenged through the BA activities scheduling

iCBT in the workplace

Alex is a 42-year-old married man who was recently promoted at work. However, in recent weeks he was beginning to feel overwhelmed. He had been working towards this promotion for years, but the reality of the extra workload and responsibility was suddenly sinking in. Alex realised he needed help when he snapped aggressively at a colleague one day; this was completely out of character for him. A few days later, a presentation was given to his department about the company's new online self-help stress programme as part of the employee assistance programme. Alex decided to give it a try since the flexibility of the intervention and its discreetness appealed to him – he could use it on his phone on the train to work and nobody would need to know.

During the programme, Alex learned problem-solving strategies through interactive activities, which helped him to deal with some matters that emerged from the new tasks. He was surprised when the programme made him aware, after completing an activity about rating the importance of time spent in different life areas, that he was prioritising his work over his family. He also learned how to challenge his distress-promoting thinking and develop techniques to use when he felt irritable or anxious. In particular, Alex uncovered a core belief about his thinking that he would not be able to cope with responsibility. Alex now recognised this core negative thought and became far better equipped to handle his new position at work – he had the tools he needed to understand when he was getting stressed and to deal with it effectively.

Self-referred iCBT

Michelle is a 19-year-old college student. She has been suffering from a steady state of worry and irritability. Her main worries are about the possibility of failing the exams, losing her friends, as well as the health of her parents, who live far away in another city. This excessive worry caused her muscular tension, hyperventilating and sleep problems. As a result, she developed safety behaviours, such as spending the whole weekend studying, offering her summaries to her friends to 'compensate for' her absence, and calling her parents every day to check up on them. Michelle felt overwhelmed by all these 'responsibilities', and she became unhappy. She saw an advertisement about online treatment for anxiety difficulties and she decided to give it a try.

She conducted a phone interview with a clinical psychologist, who diagnosed her generalised anxiety disorder (GAD), and she was offered access to an online programme specifically created to address this condition. She learned about the worry cycle through diagrams and quizzes, and this helped her to understand the benefits she was getting from worrying and the role that safety behaviours were playing in the maintenance of her disorder. Mindfulness exercises helped her not to respond to her thoughts, but to accept them and change the focus to the present. She realised how her anxiety symptoms decreased over time when looking at the mood chart after a few weeks. Through interactive tools, such as the worry tree, the programme taught her strategies for managing her worries, and she stopped using the safety behaviours, which gave her a great sense of freedom.

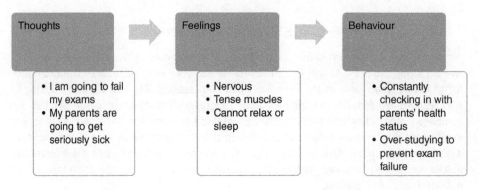

Figure 12.2   Michelle's maintaining cycle of worry in GAD

iCBT for long-term conditions

James, a 60-year-old self-employed carpenter, has been suffering from chronic lower back pain since a building site accident 20 years ago. He has increasingly struggled to meet the physical demands of his job and also feels that his pain has prevented him from spending quality time with his grandchildren. At a routine visit, James's GP noticed his low mood, irritability and pessimism about his pain, and suggested that he may benefit from therapy.

James was sceptical at first about the iCBT intervention that his therapist offered, especially as he had limited computer abilities. James was aware that he was avoiding engaging with life activities due to his pain but using the iCBT programme enabled James to see that his avoidant behaviour was a direct result of thinking and feeling about his pain and its management. Learning how to challenge his cognitions helped James to reassess his black-and-white thinking that pain equated to having to avoid pleasurable activities, such as playing with his grandchildren. James began some behavioural experiments to assess where he was comfortable in playing with his grandkids and where he needed to stop to mind himself. The iCBT programme also gave him some techniques for relaxation and meditation to help with his self-management. This new-found knowledge and strategies allowed him to re-engage in the things he enjoyed while respecting his own limitations. In addition, for James, the anonymity that iCBT afforded and the 24-hour access to his account were noted advantages.

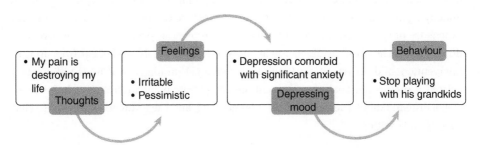

Figure 12.3   James's experience cycle

PRACTITIONER TAKE HOME MESSAGES

- iCBT has a strong empirical base
- iCBT can be implemented flexibly in a wide variety of contexts
- iCBT offers great potential for the dissemination of evidence-based treatments
- iCBT has many significant benefits for service users

Table 12.2   Thoughts, feelings and behaviour (TFB) cycle for James

	CBT Core Concepts & Processes		
	Understanding CBT model	**Behavioural activation processes**	**Cognitive processes**
iCBT platform provision of CBT using interactive tools and exercises	Slideshow on CBT model	Interactive exercise to develop behavioural experiments to help assess strengths and comfort levels	Slideshow of typical negative automatic thoughts (NATs)
	Educational video on relationship between chronic pain and comorbid anxiety and depression feelings and the application of CBT for successful management		The behavioural experiments also support challenging his negative thought that he cannot do anything because of his pain

CONCLUSION

State-of-the-art research in iCBT is encouraging, and empirical support is swelling, especially for depression and anxiety disorders, leading us to be realistic in predicting new breakthroughs on the horizon. Blended approaches to care can support the use of iCBT in more severe, enduring and complex mental health problems. We know very little about the underlying mechanisms of change in iCBT. The more we can delve into the psychological experience of service users and clinicians, the more we can develop more effective solutions. There has been some discussion about who is most suitable to benefit from an iCBT intervention, and yet our understanding of individual profiling for iCBT is rudimentary. Related is the field of adapting interventions for specific populations and cultures to aid global dissemination. The field of iCBT is burgeoning, and the future for iCBT is both challenging and exciting.

DISCUSSION QUESTIONS

1.   What are the key conclusions from the literature on using iCBT treatments?
2.   What are the main advantages and disadvantages of iCBT?
3.   How would a mental health service incorporate iCBT into their day-to-day practice?
4.   What are some important applications of iCBT in the workplace?

KEY TERMS

Cognitive Behaviour Therapy (CBT) An evidence-based, empirically supported, time-limited, structured, goal-oriented psychotherapy focused towards solving current problems and educating service users in essential skills to alter dysfunctional thinking and behaviour.

Internet-delivered cognitive behaviour therapy (iCBT) A method for the dissemination of CBT. iCBT is a repurposing of an evidence-based CBT treatment protocol into an online environment and is used in a self-administered manner, either with or without support.

Service users Clients and patients. We use the generic term to refer to all potential users of iCBT interventions.

Supporter A generic term used to describe the variety of persons that can offer guidance and support to service users as they progress through an iCBT intervention. These can include a range of health professionals, clinicians, nurse practitioners, trained volunteers and peer mentors.

─────────────────── **FURTHER READING** ───────────────────

- Andersson, G. (2014) *The internet and CBT: A clinical guide.* Boca Raton, FL: CRC Press.
- Lindefors, N. & Andersson A. (2016) *Guided internet-based treatments in psychiatry.* Cham, Switzerland: Springer.

REFERENCES

Aardoom, J. J., Dingemans, A. E., Spinhoven, P., & Van Furth, E. F. (2013) Treating eating disorders over the internet: A systematic review and future research directions. *International Journal of Eating Disorders*, *46*(6), 539–552.

American Psychiatric Association (APA) (2000) *Diagnostic and statistical manual of mental disorders: DSM-IV-TR.* Washington, DC: American Psychiatric Association.

Andersson, G. (2014) *The internet and CBT: A clinical guide.* Boca Raton, FL: CRC Press.

Andersson, G. (2016) Internet-delivered psychological treatments. *Annual Review of Clinical Psychology*, *12*, 157–179.

Andersson, G., Waara, J., Jonsson, U., Malmaeus, F., Carlbring, P., & Ost, L.-G. (2009) Internet-based self-help versus one-session exposure in the treatment of spider phobia: A randomized controlled trial. *Cognitive Behaviour Therapy*, *38*(2), 114–120.

Andersson, G., Waara, J., Jonsson, U., Malmaeus, F., Carlbring, P., & Öst, L.-G. (2013) Internet-based exposure treatment versus one-session exposure treatment of snake phobia: A randomized controlled trial. *Cognitive Behaviour Therapy*, *42*(4), 284–291.

Cavanagh, K., Shapiro, D. A., Van Den Berg, S., Swain, S., Barkham, M., & Proudfoot, J. (2006) The effectiveness of computerized cognitive behavioural therapy in routine care. *British Journal of Clinical Psychology*, *45*(4), 499–514.

Gilbody, S., Brabyn, S., Lovell, K., Kessler, D., Devlin, T., Smith, L., Araya, R., Barkham, M., Bower, P., Cooper, C., Knowles, S., Littlewood, E., Richards, D. A., Tallon, D., White, D., Worthy, G., & REEACT collaborative. (2017) Telephone-supported computerised cognitive-behavioural therapy: REEACT-2 large-scale pragmatic randomised controlled trial. *British Journal of Psychiatry*, *210*(5), 362–367.

Hanlon, P., Daines, L., Campbell, C., McKinstry, B., Weller, D., & Pinnock, H. (2017) Telehealth interventions to support self-management of long-term conditions: A systematic metareview of diabetes, heart failure, asthma, chronic obstructive pulmonary disease, and cancer. *Journal of Medical Internet Research, 19*(5), e172.

Hedman, E., Andersson, G., Andersson, E., Ljotsson, B., Ruck, C., Asmundson, G. J., & Lindefors, N. (2011) Internet-based cognitive-behavioural therapy for severe health anxiety: Randomised controlled trial. *British Journal of Psychiatry, 198*(3), 230–236.

Hedman, E., Axelsson, E., Gorling, A., Ritzman, C., Ronnheden, M., El Alaoui, S., Andersson, E., Lekander, M., & Ljotsson, B. (2014) Internet-delivered exposure-based cognitive-behavioural therapy and behavioural stress management for severe health anxiety: Randomised controlled trial. *British Journal of Psychiatry, 205*(4), 307–314.

Hollon, S. D. & Beck, A. T. (2016) Cognitive and cognitive-behavioral therapies. In M. J. Lambert (Ed.), *Handbook of psychotherapy and behavior change* (6th ed.). Hoboken, NJ: Wiley, pp. 393–394.

Johansson, R. & Andersson, G. (2012) Internet-based psychological treatments for depression. *Expert Review of Neurotherapy, 12*(7), 861–870.

Kampmann, I. L., Emmelkamp, P. M., & Morina, N. (2016). Meta-analysis of technology-assisted interventions for social anxiety disorder. *J Anxiety Disord, 42*, 71–84.

Karyotaki, E., Riper, H., Twisk, J., Hoogendoorn, A., Kleiboer, A., Mira, A., Mackinnon, A., Meyer, B., Botella, C., Littlewood, E., Andersson, G., Christensen, H., Klein, J. P., Schroder, J., Breton-Lopez, J., Scheider, J., Griffiths, K., Farrer, L., Huibers, M. J., Phillips, R., Gilbody, S., Moritz, S., Berger, T., Pop, V., Spek, V., & Cuijpers, P. (2017) Efficacy of self-guided internet-based cognitive behavioral therapy in the treatment of depressive symptoms: A meta-analysis of individual participant data. *JAMA Psychiatry, 74*(4), 351–359.

Kuester, A., Niemeyer, H., & Knaevelsrud, C. (2015) Internet-based interventions for post-traumatic stress: A meta-analysis of randomized controlled trials. *Clinical Psychology Review, 43*, 1–16.

Olthuis, J. V., Watt, M. C., Bailey, K., Hayden, J. A., & Stewart, S. H. (2016) Therapist-supported internet cognitive behavioural therapy for anxiety disorders in adults. *Cochrane Database of Systematic Reviews, 3*.

Pasarelu, C. R., Andersson, G., Bergman Nordgren, L., & Dobrean, A. (2017) Internet-delivered transdiagnostic and tailored cognitive behavioral therapy for anxiety and depression: A systematic review and meta-analysis of randomized controlled trials. *Cognitive Behaviour Therapy, 46*(1), 1–28.

Richards, D. & Richardson, T. (2012) Computer-based psychological treatments for depression: A systematic review and meta-analysis. *Clinical Psychology Review, 32*(4), 329–342.

Richards, D., Duffy, D., Blackburn, B., Earley, C., Enrique, A., Palacios, J., Franklin, M., Clarke, G., Sollesse, S., Connell, S., & Timulak, L. (2018) Digital IAPT: The effectiveness and cost-effectiveness of internet-delivered interventions for depression and anxiety disorders in the Improving Access to Psychological Therapies programme: Study protocol for a randomised control trial. *BMC Psychiatry*.

Richards, D., Richardson, T., Timulak, L. & McElvaney, J. (2015) The efficacy of internet-delivered treatment for generalized anxiety disorder: A systematic review and meta-analysis. *Internet Interventions*, *2*(3), 272–282.

Richards, D., Timulak, L., O'Brien, E., Hayes, C., Vigano, N., Sharry, J., & Doherty, G. (2015) A randomized controlled trial of an internet-delivered treatment: Its potential as a low-intensity community intervention for adults with symptoms of depression. *Behaviour Research Therapy*, *75*, 20–31.

Salamanca, A., Richards, D., Timulak, L., Castro, L., Mojica, M., & Parra, Y. (2018) Assessing the efficacy of a culturally adapted cognitive behavioural internet-delivered treatment for depression: Protocol for a randomised controlled trial. *BMC Psychiatry*.

Selmi, P. M., Klein, M. H., Greist, J. H., Sorrell, S. P., & Erdman, H. P. (1990) Computer-administered cognitive-behavioral therapy for depression. *The American Journal of Psychiatry*, *147*(1), 51–56.

Titov, N., Andrews, G., Davies, M., McIntyre, K., Robinson, E., & Solley, K. (2010) Internet treatment for depression: A randomized controlled trial comparing clinician vs. technician assistance. *PLoS ONE*, *5*(6), e10939.

Titov, N., Dear, B., Nielssen, O., Staples, L., Hadjistavropoulos, H., Nugent, M., . . . Kaldo, V. (2018). ICBT in routine care: A descriptive analysis of successful clinics in five countries. *Internet Interventions*, *13*, 108–115.

Todd, N. J., Jones, S. H., Hart, A., & Lobban, F. A. (2014) A web-based self-management intervention for bipolar disorder 'Living with Bipolar': A feasibility randomised controlled trial. *Journal of Affective Disorder*, *169*, 21–29.

van Beugen, S., Ferwerda, M., Hoeve, D., Rovers, M. M., Spillekom-van Koulil, S., van Middendorp, H., & Evers, A. W. (2014) Internet-based cognitive behavioral therapy for patients with chronic somatic conditions: A meta-analytic review. *Journal of Medical Internet Research*, *16*(3), e88.

Wells, M. J., Owen, J. J., McCray, L. W., Bishop, L. B., Ells, T. D., Brown, G. K., Richards, D., Thase, M. E., & Wright, J. H. (2018) Computer-assisted cognitive-behavior therapy for depression in primary care: Systematic review and meta-analysis. *Primary Care Companion to the Journal of Clinical Psychiatry*.

Wilson, G. T. & Zandberg, L. J. (2012) Cognitive-behavioral guided self-help for eating disorders: Effectiveness and scalability. *Clinical Psychology Review*, *32*(4), 343–357.

Wootton, B. M., Andersson, E., & Rück, C. (2016) Internet-delivered cognitive behavior therapy (iCBT) for obsessive-compulsive disorder. In N. Lindefors & G. Andersson (Eds.), *Guided internet-based treatments in psychiatry*. Champaign, IL: Springer, pp. 101–119.

Wright, J. H., Owen, J.J., Richards, D., Ells, T.D., Richardson, T., Brown, G.K., Barrett, M., Rasku, M.A., Polser, G., & Thase, M. (in press) Computer-assisted cognitive-behavior therapy for depression: A systematic review and meta-analysis. *Journal of Clinical Psychiatry*.

Wright, J. H., Eells, T., Gopalraj, R., & Bishop, L. (2018). Computer-assisted cognitive-behavior therapy in medical care settings. *Current Psychiatry Reports*, *20*, 92.

13

PSYCHOEDUCATION

SIMONE BOL

INTRODUCTION

Psychoeducation aims to provide clients and their networks with relevant and helpful information about physiological and psychological aspects of their experiences. It is used to help clients with a wide variety of psychological difficulties, as well as their support system, to understand their needs and empower their capacity to improve their wellbeing. Most psychological individual or group interventions, including Cognitive Behavioural Therapy (CBT) and Compassion Focused Therapy (CFT), contain an element of psychoeducation. Psychoeducation can also be a primary, stand-alone intervention. It can take many different forms, ranging from providing information in leaflets or via apps, to psychoeducation groups and individual sessions. Its application and use have expanded rapidly over the past few decades.

This chapter will:

- discuss how psychoeducation is used in interventions and how it can benefit clients' wellbeing through dispelling myths and empowering clients with information
- consider how psychoeducation can fit in various approaches to therapeutic work
- look at some potential challenges to using psychoeducation.

This chapter aims to:

- set out a broad overview of psychoeducation as a form of intervention
- introduce readers to a diverse range of research findings and theoretical insights relevant to psychoeducation
- provide initial practical guidance on delivering psychoeducation in therapeutic settings.

BACKGROUND

Psychoeducation's focus on providing information and skills about a client's condition or experiences makes it an easily accessible intervention. It can also be useful for clients who may not access other mental health services for fear of stigma (Cuijpers, 1998). Increasing knowledge of psychological difficulties has important therapeutic potential in itself. For instance, with understanding, there is often a clarity that emerges for clients, and this can enhance self-acceptance and self-compassion and can counteract societal stigma of mental health conditions (see, for example, DeLucia-Waack, 2006). It can provide a space for 'why is this happening?' questions. Even if there are no answers to all the 'why' questions, discussion clarifies that the client is not to blame for their symptoms. By considering clients' experiences in dialogue with a mental health practitioner and/or (expert-by-experience) peers, psychoeducation can elaborate clients' understanding of their experiences and needs, facilitating the development of expertise of their own particular experiences.

As described by Authier (1977), psychoeducation originally emerged as a response to the increase in community care, with an emphasis on providing skills and understanding for families of clients with a diagnosis of 'schizophrenia', a diagnostic term that is currently under review. Psychoeducation generally views families and support networks as potentially important resources to improve wellbeing (Walsh, 2010). Psychoeducation is a strengths- and competence-based approach (Lukens & McFarlane, 2004), which means that it focuses on recognising and developing capacities for self-care and self-advocacy in clients and their support systems. For example, psychoeducation for a client's support network can help it to be as supportive as possible due to increased knowledge and understanding about the nature of the needs, behaviours and experiences of the client. Understanding what is going on and what might be helpful for a loved one can also help to alleviate a sense of guilt, irritation or isolation that people interacting with the client in everyday life may experience (see, for example, Tanriverdi & Ekinci, 2012).

Psychoeducation is used by a wide variety of mental health practitioners from different professional backgrounds and with different therapeutic approaches (Economou, 2015). This also means that the word 'psychoeducation' is used for a wide range of activities with varying aims, also depending on the practitioner's stance on mental health difficulties and professional practice. Psychoeducation can entail providing information to convince clients of the information that practitioners feel is relevant, for example, to enhance therapy compliance or help-seeking behaviours. Other practitioners might see psychoeducation as a dialogic method to gain information from the client and facilitate the client's development of gaining understanding. Methods of delivery range from signposting to websites, providing leaflets and books ('bibliotherapy'), generally delivering 'passive psychoeducation' whereby content is fixed and provided without participation from clients, to more interactive apps and face-to-face contact, in which clients can participate in group discussions, sharing experiences or solving problems together, and may do a variety of exercises and learn coping skills (Walsh, 2010).

Psychoeducation can be delivered to individuals or groups of clients with similar needs, such as adults or children experiencing anxiety or low mood, but also to those with psychological needs in relation to living with medical conditions, such as life after a heart attack or living with persistent pain. This can be done in parallel with teaching coping techniques that are often associated with grounding or focused attention, such as teaching relaxation and mindfulness techniques (Walsh, 2010). Techniques and information might be aimed at coping with existing difficulties or preventing the emergence of difficulties, for example, providing separating parents with information and skills about healthy communication for their children. Stand-alone psychoeducation interventions can be manualised, which can also aid quantitative effectiveness and feasibility studies. For example, Mayor et al. (2013) describe how short, manualised psychoeducation can be delivered by medical staff with limited psychological training to clients who have experienced psychogenic seizures. Other examples of manualised interventions include *Pegasus* (Gordon et al., 2015), which aims to enhance self-awareness for young people on the autistic spectrum, and the *Psychoeducation Manual for Bipolar Disorder* (Colom, Vieta, & Scott, 2006).

Psychoeducation is also an important component in a variety of broader therapeutic interventions, either in a planned or emerging-in-the-moment manner. For example, it is a crucial planned component in early interventions for people who have received a diagnosis of schizophrenia and have unusual experiences, such as hearing voices or seeing visions (Hastrup et al., 2013). Beck (1995) advises that in cognitive therapy, which he developed into CBT, educating the client to become his or her own therapist is one of the main principles of the therapy. By developing a mutual understanding of the client's experiences and making sense of these with the help of the practitioner's knowledge base, clients also gain insight into the rationales and mechanisms of the therapy process as envisaged by the practitioner. This can help clients to feel safer and more in control in the therapeutic process. The time, effort and sometimes difficult emotions that can be part of a therapeutic process are easier to tolerate when it is clear why these may occur. Shapiro (2001), in her description of the main principles of Eye Movement Desensitisation Reprocessing (EMDR) therapy, an evidence-based intervention for post-traumatic stress disorder (PTSD), also relates this increased and shared understanding to clients' ability to continue with therapy.

To conclude, psychoeducation can provide clients and their support systems with useful skills and information as well as a sense of agency, giving them the ability to influence their life and environment, and helping them to make informed choices about their lifestyle and therapeutic options. This is often hugely empowering.

PSYCHOEDUCATION EVIDENCE BASE: DOES IT WORK?

Looking at psychoeducation delivered as a stand-alone intervention for what historically has been called 'schizophrenia', many studies have confirmed its effectiveness in the short and medium term (Lukens & McFarlane, 2004; Xia, Merinder, & Belgamwar, 2011; Zhao et al., 2015). For middle- and low-income countries, Chatterjee et al. (2014)

suggest that community-delivered psychoeducation can be more effective than standard hospital procedures and is particularly relevant where services are scarce. The community-delivered care project in India that Chatterjee et al. (2014) investigated was developed in collaboration with people with schizophrenia and their families, and was delivered by community health workers with a generic education and good interpersonal skills, who were supervised by mental health social workers. There was also signposting to community and expert-by-experience self-help groups in this project. This care was found to be more effective than care delivered in a mental health facility by specialist mental health practitioners, consisting of brief consultations and medication prescription.

The evidence base for psychoeducation for common psychological difficulties, such as depression and anxiety, has significantly expanded over recent years. Tursi et al. (2013) found that a variety of psychoeducation interventions, although at times difficult to compare, proved effective in interventions for depression and anxiety. Shimazu et al. (2011) conclude that a psychoeducation programme for the relatives of people experiencing depression, providing information on the symptoms and nature of the condition as well as practical exercises facilitating family members to find their own solutions for dealing with difficult emotional situations, resulted in significantly fewer readmissions to hospital at the nine-month follow-up date. Donker et al. (2009) highlight in a meta-analysis that even brief, passive psychoeducational intervention on its own (for example, when delivered by a leaflet or an email) can provide some relief in anxiety and depression. Delivering supportive psychoeducation for carers of people with dementia has been shown to alleviate stress, improve mood and reduce anxiety for carers, and is likely to benefit the partner with dementia too (Pendergrass et al., 2015). Psychoeducation is recommended as a first step in a stepped-care approach for common mental health difficulties such as anxiety and depression. This is advocated both in the UK context and in the US (National Institute for Clinical Excellence, 2011; O'Donohue & Draper, 2011). Burns, Kellett and Donohue (2016) looked at psychoeducation as Step 2 of a common care pathway in the UK, as recommended by NICE (2011), which focuses on stress control for clients with mild mood and anxiety disorders. The sessions focused on providing information about the neurophysiology of stress, exercises to help control stress, and included topics about sleep and self-care. Burns et al. (2016) found that this psychoeducational intervention proved effective for a high proportion of the participants, particularly for those who attended all six sessions of the intervention.

Dropout rates are important when considering effectiveness. Burns et al. (2016) found the highest dropout rates in participants living in areas of greater deprivation. Cuijpers et al. (2010) conclude that passive self-help therapy overall has a similar dropout rate to face-to-face therapy, but they note that clients probably self-select a method that suits them. Offering clients a range of options can facilitate uptake. Baillie and Rapee (2004) and Haug et al. (2015) looked into predicting who might benefit from psychoeducation for panic disorders most and found that clients without additional social fear or profound mental health difficulties were more likely to recover through a psychoeducation programme as a stand-alone intervention.

It is also important to consider whether there can be reasons why psychoeducation programmes may be unhelpful in some instances. Wesseley et al. (2008) discuss that providing information about PTSD to people who have experienced a trauma can establish unhelpful and unwarranted negative expectations, and at times information contains advice that undermines people's own instinctual coping mechanisms.

Overall, it can be concluded that many systematic reviews provide evidence for the usefulness of psychoeducation using particular programmes and for specific populations. However, effectiveness can be improved further when more is learned about what precisely works best and what might work less well for others (see also Donker et al., 2009; Xia et al., 2011; Grácio, Gonçalves-Pereira, & Leff, 2015).

THEORETICAL INSIGHTS INTO PSYCHOEDUCATION

The content of psychoeducation programmes varies, and particular exercises and content may be more or less effective. What can be said about the process of psychoeducation in general, though? What general mechanisms are likely to make psychoeducation work? Here I will discuss the communicative processes involved in psychoeducation, including providing advice, the use of language and providing symbolic resources for externalisation and new narratives, and social support and power relations.

Many studies show that providing advice that is not developed in collaboration with the client is far less likely to be successfully implemented (see discussions in Couture & Sutherland, 2006; and Ekberg & LeCouteur, 2013). Taking this evidence into account, psychoeducation that is to some degree tailored to the individual needs of the client may have advantages over a highly structured and standardised package, in some instances. It is also important to look at the content of standardised programmes and how language and concepts are used in relation to the client's needs and context. Wilson et al. (2018) discuss how a text for a standardised psychoeducation programme for bipolar disorder contains a lot of language that, in their opinion, could be perceived as disempowering, or potentially even demeaning. The language used in programmes needs to align to the client's context and the practitioner's perspective on empowering language use. Psychoeducation can be conceptualised as a space in which new narratives and perspectives can be formed, often in supportive dialogue with a practitioner, family members and/or peers.

Larsen's (2007) in-depth ethnographic study of psychoeducation groups demonstrates how language and symbolic resources, such as concepts about heritability, can be more or less useful resources for participants in a psychoeducation programme. He distinguishes words that relate to an 'illness identity', referring to who a person 'is' and 'will be', and words relating to an 'illness experience', which allows for change and recovery. Therefore, some concepts and words are likely to be more empowering than others. The symbolisation process in psychoeducation provided some clients with a space to look at their experiences anew and supported them in creating a story as part of their recovery process. It 'dedramatised' the experience, allowing some clients to stop blaming themselves. This use of symbolic resources to create a new narrative is in line with the concept of 'externalising', as used in social constructionist narrative approaches. White and Epston (1990) explore how this process allows clients to view an aspect of themselves in a different light and allows clients to create a new story of themselves with this new configuration. McLeod (1997) emphasises that shame can silence and prevent people from even thinking about their own story, and it is easy to see how supportive psychoeducation, for example with a peer group and/or from an expert patient who has a similar experience, can provide an excellent platform for new narratives. In dialogues and group dynamics, power relations impact how symbolic resources are negotiated. In this respect, Burman (2016) maintains that good psychoeducation needs to be 'didactic but not directive', and that the common humanity of the practitioner and client need to be attended to in order for psychoeducation to be truly empowering.

PRACTICAL POINTS

Psychoeducation can take many different forms and be tailored to various conditions and groups of people, so practicalities and required skills vary. What is clear is that the communication with the client is important in order for clients to be able to benefit. In this section, various practical aspects that apply to delivering many psychoeducational interventions will be discussed.

PSYCHOEDUCATION AND RELATIONSHIPS

In many mental health difficulties, confusion, shame and anxiety play a role, and are potentially related to stigma and/or the condition itself. Practitioners providing psycho education need to consider the evidence base for a positive therapeutic alliance in order to provide an optimal environment for learning and change (Levy-Frank et al., 2012). Depending on the mode of delivery, and the therapeutic model used, some authors argue that coaching, group leader or teaching skills are more salient in psychoeducation (see, for example, DeLucia-Waack, 2006; Walsh, 2010; Brown, 2011). Practitioners using a humanistic model are likely to focus on establishing a genuine relationship and wanting to hear the meanings that experiences have for clients, whereas practitioners acting from a medical stance may put more emphasis on providing information. Group settings and working with children may require more explicit boundary and rule setting, whereas individual psychoeducation with adults may look more collegiate.

When working with family groups, the practitioner's views on family communications need to be taken into account. Walsh (2010) discusses how practitioners can coach communication between family members, for example by supporting a family member with mental health difficulties to share their experiences and needs. Involving skilled service users and peers in psychoeducation can provide clients with positive relationships that have less of a power difference and can alleviate stigma and feelings of being alone.

When delivering psychoeducation in groups, paying attention to the normal anxiety of starting in a group, for example by providing ice breakers, setting clear rules and proving a reliable setting, are likely to make the group much more effective (DeLucia-Waack, 2006; Walsh, 2010). Helping clients to find similarities and recognition to allow for initial social support can also be useful. These similarities can initially be around trivial matters, but towards the middle of an initial setting it is, in my experience, useful to facilitate the sharing of more serious aspects that tie in to the aims of the group. This allows the group to be a space where something useful can be found for participants and openness about difficulties has a place. Focusing on similarities as well as differences can facilitate an accepting and open atmosphere.

PSYCHOEDUCATION AND LEARNING PROCESSES

Reducing anxiety as well as valuing and re-activating someone's existing knowledge aids information processing (Jarvis, 2010). For example, by asking questions in a way that emphasises an interest in people's own experiences, rather than their general knowledge about a topic, anxiety can be reduced as there is no right or wrong answer. It activates the memory of an experience and expresses that the person's life experiences are important to consider.

Emotional distress often impacts upon people's ability to concentrate, remember and attend to information (Fine, 2008). Simple measures, such as using short sentences, providing written or other visual aids that can be looked at again, and paraphrasing information, can be helpful when delivering psychoeducation. Particularly in adult education, it is important to value people's existing knowledge, and previous positive and negative experiences, with training and education (Jarvis, 2010). Information needs to be clear and accessible, but not patronising.

Metaphors are often used to explain something in a vivid and entertaining way. Visual representation may help those with limited attention spans or a preference for visual representations. Metaphors can bridge one domain, the mental health difficulties, with another domain, of experience and the concepts that the client is already familiar with, and can communicate something of the emotional load of the experience too (Stott, 2010). For example, metaphors such as 'a storm in your head', describing fast and relentless thoughts, can also signify unpredictability and an experience of threat. Creative methods and the use of objects or toys can be used as powerful metaphors and symbolic representations too (DeLucia-Waack, 2006).

TOP TIPS

Carefully consider the language used in programmes - language matters!

Symbolisation and externalisation can be powerful tools in psychoeducation - use them wisely!

Be careful around taking too much of an expert role as it can be disempowering for clients. Sharing common humanity and knowledge is always a good start.

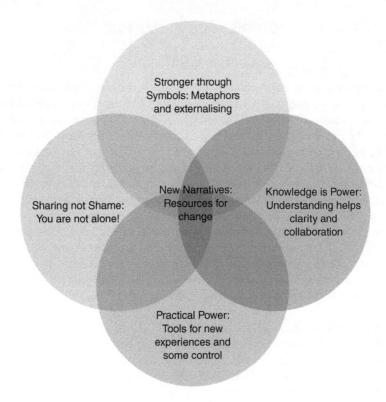

Figure 13.1 The Four Forces Model of Psychoeducation

FOUR FORCES MODEL OF PSYCHOEDUCATION

The Four Forces Model of Psychoeducation (Figure 13.1) demonstrates the potentially empowering and practical forces behind successful psychoeducation interventions. The four elements are:

1. **Stronger through Symbols**: Metaphors and externalising provide clients with tools for new narratives.
2. **Sharing not Shame**: Contact – in whatever form – with peers/practitioner/expert-client, their experiences and common humanity can provide clients with a safe social network to start seeing themselves in a different light, changing self-perceptions.
3. **Knowledge is Power**: Gaining an insight into the causes and nature of difficulties can alleviate self-blame, help reflection and externalisation and can facilitate collaboration between client and practitioner. It can help those around a client gain insight and compassion.
4. **Practical Power**: Clients gain tools to change their lives in ways that are helpful to them and alleviate distress. This also allows for new experiences that can challenge negative self-perceptions and feelings of helplessness.

The case studies below will be used to demonstrate the Four Forces Model in action.

--- STORIES FROM PRACTICE ---

Georgina: Not alone

Georgina had come to our psychotherapy service to cope better with difficulties in her every-day life related to the diagnosis Borderline Personality Disorder she had received some time before. She struggled with emotion regulation, and initially self-harmed when emotions were too intense for her. She felt a great deal of shame and responsibility about this behaviour. We discussed the function that pain and self-harm had for her in relation to emotion regulation, but only when I introduced some worksheets to help her recognise the emotional states she was experiencing, did she seem to fully appreciate that she was not alone in this experience and not the only one with these behaviours. Georgina laughed, relieved at the worksheet, and told me 'So, I am not the only looney doing these things?! Someone has actually written a book about this stuff!' There was a great sense of relief and a reduction of the shame she felt as a result of this. Using her sense of humour to refer to the social stigma allowed us to talk more freely about Georgina's often overwhelming emotions and their relationship to feeling an impulse to self-harm. This, in combination with strategies to regulate emotions, eventually helped Georgina to reduce her self-harm significantly.

- *Main Empowering Force for Georgina*: Sharing not Shame
- *Supporting Empowering Force*: Stronger through Symbols and Practical Power
- *Practical Points*: The language of the worksheet was sufficiently in tune with Georgina's experiences and helped her feel taken seriously. It was offered as a suggestion in a well-developed therapeutic alliance.

Emotional Wellbeing Group

As a brief intervention for children with mental health difficulties such as low mood, anxiety and mild levels of self-harm, Ben, an assistant psychologist, and Ciara, a clinical psychologist, ran a six-session wellbeing group based on the principles of Cognitive Behaviour Therapy: Session 1: Getting to know each other and setting ground rules; Session 2: Understanding emotions; Session 3: Thoughts in your head; Session 3: Peace and quiet; Session 4: Stress busters; Session 5: What makes me happy; and Session 6: Celebration time! Lots of discussion time, creative and active activities and attention to the children's needs helped to create a productive and supportive group. Ben and Ciara's main aim was to provide the children with strategies to self-soothe and manage their feelings and behaviours. The children had fun, but also discussed their difficulties and learned techniques from each other. Ben and Ciara were able to help the children to be aware of the thoughts that were helpful or not helpful, to recognise their emotions, and to use a range of relaxation and distraction techniques to improve their wellbeing.

- *Main Empowering Force of the Group*: Practical Power
- *Supporting Empowering Forces*: Sharing not Shame and Stronger through Symbols in creative activities (e.g. drawing their anger monsters)
- *Practical Points*: Attention to group processes and group relations. Adapting the concepts and activities to the developmental level of the children.

Halima: A new narrative

Halima came to our counselling service because she was concerned about her mental health. The same time a year before she had had to take time off work and had needed to be hospitalised due to severe depression. She was very worried about being depressed but did not experience low mood as such. The main issue for her was to make sense of what had happened, why it might have happened, and what to do if it happened again. I listened to Halima's experiences of being hospitalised and what had happened in the time leading up to her hospitalisation. Taking a largely non-directive approach initially, Halima's own story became clearer. My contributions were to reflect what had been important to her and to suggest, on a few occasions, how, in my opinion, that might have contributed to her breakdown. Halima concluded there was a bereavement process that she needed to find some closure on, and that this would be important for her mental health. She visited her aunt's grave abroad, a trip she made on her own, which was something she had not done in the past. Halima felt she understood what had happened to her, that she had been able to do something constructive about this, and that should she have a depressed episode again, she would know where to get help.

- *Main Empowering Force for Halima*: Knowledge is Power
- *Supporting Empowering Forces*: Sharing not Shame, and Halima created her own Practical Power in going on a trip as part of her bereavement process
- *Practical Points*: Attention for common humanity rather than an expert position of the therapist.

Agata's information needs

Agata, a solicitor in her 30s, had been admitted to a psychiatric intensive care unit for the first time in her life after a suicide attempt while she was on antidepressant medication. Agata presented with very rapid and associative thoughts which frightened her, and she wanted them to stop. She was also afraid that someone was trying to poison her with the antidepressants.

In her meeting with Agata, Amina, the psychiatrist, had the psychoeducational goals of explaining her new diagnosis to Agata and for Agata to trust the new medication she was prescribing. Amina felt that Agata had bipolar disorder and was currently experiencing a manic episode, probably elicited by the antidepressants. Agata's ability to attend to the information was rather limited due to the manic episode. Agata was also very upset and confused by all the thoughts in her head and her first experience of being on a psychiatric ward.

In the meeting, Amina made sure she provided Agata with an opportunity to explain her frustrations and experiences before sharing information, and she was very empathic and respectful of these, assisting the start of a trusting relationship and helping somewhat in alleviating Agata's anxiety. Amina was also able to validate Agata's experiences about the antidepressants not being good for her.

Agata left the meeting feeling very relieved, as she now felt less frightened about her rapid thoughts and she understood her felt sense of being poisoned. It was a good start of a fruitful collaboration in which Amina took Agata's needs and existing knowledge seriously. Agata was able to leave the ward in a few days, taking her new medication.

- *Main Empowering Force for Agata*: Knowledge is Power
- *Supporting Empowering Forces*: Sharing not Shame and Stronger through Symbols; the 'poisoning' started to make sense in dialogue
- *Practical Points*: Amina took Agata's information-processing difficulties (due to frustration and anxiety around being on a ward and her hypomanic state) into account and acknowledged Agata's expertise and life experience. Amina took a collaborative approach.

EVALUATION

Psychoeducation has many applications and can take different forms and directions, depending on the therapeutic stance of the practitioner. Even simple, low-cost, passive psychoeducational interventions, such as leaflets and websites, have been found to have an effect. There is evidence of the effectiveness for many programmes and many mental health conditions, but there is a need for more research into the long-term effects, and the great variety of psychoeducational applications makes systematic reviews challenging. However, there is good theoretical evidence that variation in delivery may be useful in adapting to clients' diverse needs. It is important to consider how psychoeducation may lead to practitioners taking an expert role, which can be disempowering, as well as how implicit communication is dealt with in psychoeducation. Tobias et al. (2008), coming from a Mentalization-Based Treatment (MBT) approach influenced by psychodynamic and attachment theory, warn against intellectualisation as a practitioner defence, and encourage practitioners to remain present and in tune with their own emotional processes when conducting psychoeducation. At times, practitioners might be attracted to going into 'lecturing mode' when the anxiety of 'not knowing' might be too hard to deal with (see, for example, Hansen, 1997). Psychoeducation has the strong potential of being useful, empowering and supportive of therapeutic collaboration. At the surface, the approach is often simple. Still, there are many aspects to consider that underpin the often profound effects and effectiveness of psychoeducation.

─────────────── DISCUSSION QUESTIONS ───────────────

1. What do you consider to be the advantages and disadvantages of structured programmes?
2. How does psychoeducation fit in with your philosophy of practice?
3. What do you consider to be the important skills for a practitioner providing psychoeducation?

─────────────────── KEY TERMS ───────────────────

Psychoeducation A psychosocial intervention aiming to provide clients and/or their network with a greater understanding of their physical and/or psychological difficulties and needs, empowering clients to make informed choices to enhance their wellbeing.

Support system or network Peers, friends, family, professionals or other people who are important to the client.

FURTHER READING

- DeLucia-Waack, J. L. (2006). *Leading psychoeducational groups for children and adoles-cents*. London: Sage. This publication is particularly useful when considering HOW to do psychoeducation. This is a very practical book, providing a good insight into the many different skills that practitioners need to develop when running psychoeducational groups for children and young people. It is based on the guidelines of the (American) Association for Specialists in Group Work, so – as is expected of a book that describes practicalities – it takes a particular stance on psychoeducation.
- Lukens, E. & McFarlane, W. (2004). Psychoeducation as evidence-based practice: Considerations for practice, research, and policy. *Brief Treatment and Crisis Intervention*, 4(3), 205-225. This publication is particularly useful when considering WHY to do psychoeducation. This frequently cited article reviews 16 randomised control trials investigating a breadth of applications of psychoeducation, including mental and physical health. Reading this article will provide the reader with a thorough overview of a range of applications and their effectiveness. It takes a quantitative stance on evaluating effectiveness.
- Walsh, J. (2010). *Psychoeducation in mental health*. Chicago, IL: Lyceum Books. This book is particularly useful when considering WHAT psychoeducation can be about. It provides an accessible and practical overview of psychoeducation with a US focus. It includes a brief overview of how psychoeducation is viewed from different theoretical positions. Walsh then briefly describes a range of mental health difficulties, including eating disorders, substance abuse and disruptive behaviour disorders, outlines risk and resilience factors and then provides an overview of psychoeducational programmes and relevant content.

REFERENCES

Authier, J. (1977). The psychoeducation model: Definition, contemporary roots and content. *Canadian Journal of Counselling and Psychotherapy*, 1(17).

Baillie, A. & Rapee, R. (2004). Predicting who benefits from psychoeducation and self-help for panic attacks. *Behaviour Research and Therapy*, 42(5), 513–527.

Beck, J. (1995). *Cognitive therapy*. New York: Guilford Press.

Brown, N. (2011). *Psychoeducational groups: Process and practice*. Hove: Routledge.

Burman, E. (2016). Fanon, Foucault, feminisms: Psychoeducation, theoretical psychology, and political change. *Theory & Psychology*, 26(6), 706–730.

Burns, P., Kellett, S., & Donohoe, G. (2016). 'Stress control' as a large group psycho educational intervention at Step 2 of IAPT services: Acceptability of the approach and moderators of effectiveness. *Behavioural and Cognitive Psychotherapy*, 44(4), 431–443.

Chatterjee, S., Naik, S., John, S., Dabholkar, H., Balaji, M., Koschorke, M., Varghese, M., Thara, R., Weiss, H., Williams, P., McCrone, P., Patel, V., & Thornicroft, G. (2014). Effectiveness of a community-based intervention for people with schizophrenia and their caregivers in India (COPSI): A randomised controlled trial. *The Lancet*, 383(9926), 1385–1394.

Colom, F., Vieta, E., & Scott, J. (2006). *Psychoeducation manual for bipolar disorder.* Cambridge: Cambridge University Press.

Couture, S. & Sutherland, O. (2006). Giving advice on advice-giving: A conversational analysis of Karl Tomm's practice. *Journal of Marital and Family Therapy, 32*(3), 329–344.

Cuijpers, P. (1998). A psychoeducational approach to the treatment of depression: A meta-analysis of Lewinsohn's 'coping with depression' course. *Behavior Therapy, 29*(3), 521–533.

Cuijpers, P., Donker, T., van Straten, A., Li, J., & Andersson, G. (2010). Is guided self-help as effective as face-to-face psychotherapy for depression and anxiety disorders? A systematic review and meta-analysis of comparative outcome studies. *Psychological Medicine, 40*(12), 1943–1957.

DeLucia-Waack, J. L. (2006). *Leading psychoeducational groups for children and adolescents.* London: Sage.

Donker, T., Griffiths, K., Cuijpers, P., & Christensen, H. (2009). Psychoeducation for depression, anxiety and psychological distress: A meta-analysis. *BMC Medicine, 7*(1).

Economou, M. (2015). Psychoeducation: A multifaceted intervention. *International Journal of Mental Health, 44*(4), 259–262.

Ekberg, K. & LeCouteur, A. (2013). Co-implicating and re-shaping clients' suggestions for behavioural change in cognitive behavioural therapy practice. *Qualitative Research in Psychology, 11*(1), 60–77.

Fine, J. (2008). *Language in psychiatry.* London: Equinox.

Gordon, K., Murin, M., Baykaner, O., Roughan, L., Livermore-Hardy, V., Skuse, D., & Mandy, W. (2015). A randomised controlled trial of PEGASUS, a psychoeducational programme for young people with high-functioning autism spectrum disorder. *Journal of Child Psychology and Psychiatry, 56*(4), 468–476.

Grácio, J., Gonçalves-Pereira, M., & Leff, J. (2015). What do we know about family interventions for psychosis at the process level? A systematic review. *Family Process, 55*(1), 79–90.

Hansen, J. T. (1997). The counseling process and the management of countertransference anxiety with disturbed clients. *Journal of Mental Health Counseling, 19*(4), 364–372.

Hastrup, L., Kronborg, C., Bertelsen, M., Jeppesen, P., Jorgensen, P., Petersen, L., Thorup, A., Simonsen, E., & Nordentoft, M. (2013). Cost-effectiveness of early intervention in first-episode psychosis: Economic evaluation of a randomised controlled trial (the OPUS study). *The British Journal of Psychiatry, 202*(1), 35–41.

Haug, T., Nordgreen, T., Öst, L., Kvale, G., Tangen, T., Andersson, G., Carlbring, P., Heiervang, E., & Havik, O. (2015). Stepped care versus face-to-face cognitive behavior therapy for panic disorder and social anxiety disorder: Predictors and moderators of outcome. *Behaviour Research and Therapy, 71*, 76–89.

Jarvis, P. (2010). *Adult education and lifelong learning.* Abingdon: Routledge.

Larsen, J. (2007). Symbolic healing of early psychosis: Psychoeducation and sociocultural processes of recovery. *Culture, Medicine and Psychiatry*, *31*(3), 283–306.

Levy-Frank, I., Hasson-Ohayon, I., Kravetz, S., & Roe, D. (2012). A narrative evaluation of a psychoeducation and a therapeutic alliance intervention for parents of persons with a severe mental illness. *Family Process*, *51*(2), 265–280.

Lukens, E. & McFarlane, W. (2004). Psychoeducation as evidence-based practice: Considerations for practice, research, and policy. *Brief Treatment and Crisis Intervention*, *4*(3), 205–225.

Mayor, R., Brown, R., Cock, H., House, A., Howlett, S., Smith, P., & Reuber, M. (2013). A feasibility study of a brief psycho-educational intervention for psychogenic nonepileptic seizures. *Seizure*, *22*(9), 760–765.

McLeod, J. (1997). *Narrative and psychotherapy*. London: Sage.

National Institute for Clinical Excellence (2011). *Common mental health problems: Identification and pathways to care*. Clinical Guideline 123. London: NICE. Available at: www.nice.org.uk/guidance/cg123.

O'Donohue, W. & Draper, C. (2011). *Stepped care and e-health*. New York: Springer.

Pendergrass, A., Clemens Becker, C., Hautzinger, M., & Pfeiffer, K. (2015). Dementia caregiver interventions: A systematic review of caregiver outcomes and instruments in randomized controlled trials. *International Journal of Emergency Mental Health and Human Resilience*, *17*(2), 459–468.

Shapiro, F. (2001). *Eye movement desensitization and reprocessing*. New York: Guilford Press.

Shimazu, K., Shimodera, S., Mino, Y., Nishida, A., Kamimura, N., Sawada, K., Fujita, H., Furukawa, T., & Inoue, S. (2011). Family psychoeducation for major depression: Randomised controlled trial. *The British Journal of Psychiatry*, *198*(5), 385–390.

Stott, R. (2010). *Oxford guide to metaphors in CBT*. Oxford: Oxford University Press.

Tanriverdi, D. & Ekinci, M. (2012). The effect psychoeducation intervention has on the caregiving burden of caregivers for schizophrenic patients in Turkey. *International Journal of Nursing Practice*, *18*(3), 281–288.

Tobias, G., Haslam-Hopwood, G., Allen, J., Stein, A., & Bleiberg, E. (2008). Enhancing mentalizing through psycho-education. In J. Allen & P. Fonagy (Eds.), *The handbook of mentalization-based treatment*. Chichester: John Wiley & Sons, pp. 249–268.

Tursi, M., Baes, C., Camacho, F., Tofoli, S., & Juruena, M. (2013). Effectiveness of psychoeducation for depression: A systematic review. *Australian & New Zealand Journal of Psychiatry*, *47*(11), 1019–1031.

Walsh, J. (2010). *Psychoeducation in mental health*. Chicago, IL: Lyceum Books.

Wesseley, S., Bryant, R., Greenberg, N., Earnshaw, M., Sharpley, J., & Hughes, J. (2008). Does psychoeducation help prevent post-traumatic psychological distress? *Psychiatry: Interpersonal and Biological Processes*, *71*(4), 287–302.

White, M. & Epston, D. (1990). *Narrative means to therapeutic ends*. Adelaide: Dulwich Centre.

Wilson, L., Crowe, M., Scott, A., & Lacey, C. (2018). Psychoeducation for bipolar disorder: A discourse analysis. *International Journal of Mental Health Nursing, 27*(1): 349–357.

Xia, J., Merinder, L. B., & Belgamwar, M. R. (2011). Psychoeducation for schizophrenia. *Cochrane Database of Systematic Reviews,* 6.

Zhao, S., Sampson, S., Xia, J., & Jayaram, M. B. (2015). Psychoeducation (brief) for people with serious mental illness. *Cochrane Database of Systematic Reviews,* 4.

14

INTEGRATING CORE APPROACHES

SARAH PARRY

INTRODUCTION

Throughout the book so far, the authors have introduced individual models and approaches with their particular philosophical backgrounds and techniques inherent to each modality. However, you will also have noticed many of the similarities that exist across the models and how approaches can be used together. For example, Laura Richardson explained in her chapter how art therapy has various adaptations for brief Cognitive Behavioural Therapy (CBT), Cognitive Analytic Therapy (CAT) and other models (Hughes, 2016). Similarly, I discussed how the basic principles of Motivational Interviewing (MI) make it a useful approach either before therapy starts or at the beginning of the therapeutic process. Increasingly, studies are demonstrating that including MI at the beginning of an intervention or when a client becomes stuck can significantly support the process of change in therapy (e.g. Westra & Norouzian, 2018). The Spirt of MI facilitates the development of the therapeutic relationship, empowers the client to make informed choices and identifies whether the client is ready to embark on a therapeutic journey. Lastly, Will Curvis provides a fascinating overview of how approaches can be used together in complex hospital settings (e.g. CBT, Acceptance and Commitment Therapy (ACT), mindfulness-based approaches, Solution-Focused Brief Therapy (SFBT), MI, etc.), depending upon the needs of the client and service. We have also covered some integrative models such as CBT, ACT, Compassionate Mind Training (CMT) and CAT. For many practitioners lucky enough to be trained in multiple modalities, working integratively with various techniques and approaches from across the therapeutic models becomes second nature, as getting to know the client and their formulation often highlights the need for more than one approach.

Recognising that everyone is unique and that their circumstances are often complex and multifaceted, a therapist working in an integrative way will use their knowledge of a range of models to develop a tailored therapeutic intervention for each client. Increasingly, most therapeutic practitioners (up to 85%) are now working integratively with a range of approaches (Tasca et al., 2015; Zarbo, Tasca, Cattafi, & Compare, 2016), blending them together in a complementary way for each client. For relatively recently qualified practitioners, such as myself, we have trained under a system that heavily critiques the 'deficit' model of mental health, often preferring a transdiagnostic and holistic understanding of a person's needs, strengths and difficulties. Therefore, it is perhaps not surprising that we are looking more broadly at what therapeutic modalities have to offer to our work with clients, rather than which therapeutic style fits a 'disorder'.

While the evidence base around integrative approaches continues to expand, informing practice, it is difficult to systematically review the vast range of integrative interventions in terms of their consistency or use of protocols due to factors such as individual practitioner styles, the inherent fluidity in many integrative approaches, and the gap between practice and research. Individualised, fluid, integrative approaches do not lend themselves to randomised control trial research designs, meaning that many integrative therapists rely on qualitative empirical studies, small-scale outcome studies and case studies for the evidence base. CAT is often the exception to this rule, as the CAT community has contributed heavily to the literature base, with its integrative but structured therapeutic style making systematic research and comparison to other modalities increasingly possible (see Quraishi, 2009). However, while evidence-based practice, practice guidelines and professional frameworks are important and should be an integral part of how a therapist operates, integrative therapists often recognise that the evidence base bears some biases towards particular therapeutic models that can be researched through a biomedical lens (e.g. CBT). Therapeutic integration is about drawing on the most useful and relevant components of therapeutic models to create an individualised therapeutic programme for one's clients, based on professional judgement, guidelines, expertise and formulation.

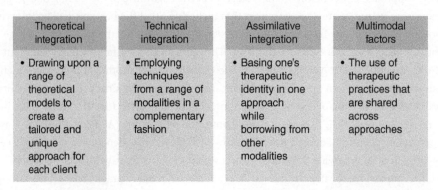

Theoretical integration	Technical integration	Assimilative integration	Multimodal factors
• Drawing upon a range of theoretical models to create a tailored and unique approach for each client	• Employing techniques from a range of modalities in a complementary fashion	• Basing one's therapeutic identity in one approach while borrowing from other modalities	• The use of therapeutic practices that are shared across approaches

Figure 14.1 The four approaches to working integratively (adapted from Castonguay et al., 2015; Kozarić-Kovacić, 2008; Zarbo et al., 2016)

THE THERAPEUTIC RELATIONSHIP IN INTEGRATIVE APPROACHES

As for all brief interventions, the therapeutic relationship is of essential importance in integrative approaches. It is generally thought to account for 30% of the therapeutic change that occurs (Lambert, 1992), while the therapeutic modality only influences around 15% of change. Mental health services that are familiar to working with integrative frameworks, such as trauma-informed services, often explicitly focus upon developing a secure base within the therapeutic relationship as a first step, before any other work can take place. Although we introduced relational commonalities that cross interventions in the introduction to this book, a recent qualitative study has highlighted six relational components that clients associate with a *healing therapeutic relationship* specifically in integrative psychotherapy (Modic & Žvelc, 2015; see Figure 14.2).

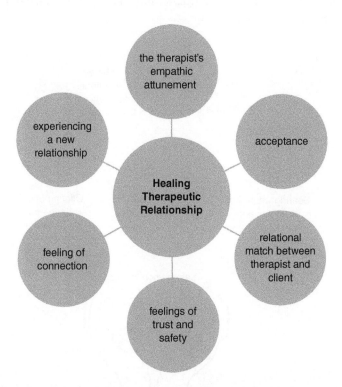

Figure 14.2 A visual representation of the healing therapeutic relationship (based on Modic & Žvelc, 2015)

These components connect closely to ideas around developing a safe base within the therapeutic relationship, as we can understand it through attachment theory (Bowlby, 1969/1982), which has also been mentioned in several of the chapters in this book.

With the growing interest in the relevance of attachment theory in adult relationships over recent years, researchers have explored the role of a secure base in therapy (e.g. Holmes, 2001; McLean, Bailey, & Lumley, 2014; Berry & Danquah, 2016) and concluded that the attachment styles of the client and therapist 'are likely to affect [the relationship's] quality, and ultimately therapeutic outcome' (Rubino, Barker, Roth, & Fearon, 2000, p. 408).

In a review a colleague and I conducted a few years ago around interventions for adult survivors of childhood sexual abuse, we consistently found that it was the experiencing of a safe, trusting, equal and respectful relationship that people identified as healing – experientially learning how it felt to be in such a relationship. It was this experiential learning through feeling that then seemed to create the platform for further therapeutic change and post-traumatic growth (Parry & Simpson, 2016). Drawing on this literature base and the original theory, Figure 14.3 can guide us in understanding more about the powerful role of a secure therapeutic relationship and its healing qualities, supporting the client in the therapeutic process.

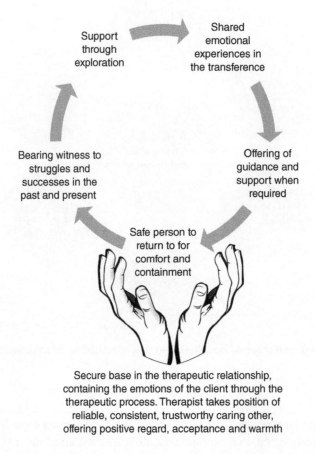

Secure base in the therapeutic relationship, containing the emotions of the client through the therapeutic process. Therapist takes position of reliable, consistent, trustworthy caring other, offering positive regard, acceptance and warmth

Figure 14.3 Illustration of the role of the therapeutic alliance through the lens of attachment theory

--- STORIES FROM PRACTICE ---

With so many options in terms of how to design and deliver integrative therapies, the following stories from practice provide ideas and insights, rather than a prescription to particular therapeutic programmes.

Ellie: Integrating compassion and reducing risk (12 sessions)

Ellie, aged 15, was referred to a young people's mental health service with a queried eating disorder (ED), as her body mass index (BMI) was only 16.5 at the point of referral. During a team meeting, it was recommended that Ellie and I would complete a Cognitive Behavioural Therapy (CBT) workbook, designed for young women with disordered eating and low self-esteem, while a specialist nurse and I monitored her weight and diet. This approach adhered to practice guidelines.

During our two initial assessment sessions, a collaborative risk management plan was developed between Ellie, her mother, the nurse and I. Throughout this time, I began to understand how early attachment losses and modelled behaviours at home had led to the development of low self-esteem and self-critical obsessive thoughts. I hypothesised how these early experiences were connected to Ellie's current relationship with herself and food.

Accordingly, I re-examined the professional guidelines and proposed an alternative intervention, including CBT and elements of Compassionate-Focused Therapy. I discussed this approach with Ellie and her mother, who were in favour of this new direction. They agreed that I could share information around Ellie's weight gain or loss with the nurse to ensure the consistent management of this specific risk to Ellie's physical health, which the nurse reported as a helpful process to her decision-making and care coordination.

Over the following sessions, we explored Ellie's self-talk and how it was connected to the language bullies had used at school, which she had internalised. Drawing on Ellie's enjoyment of art (and fantastic stationery!), we drew out the common phrases and words in the self-talk (e.g. *not tall enough, not pretty enough, stupid*) and passed them through a metaphorical mirror, turning them from critical to compassionate statements about herself. Additionally, Ellie described herself as a 'perfectionist', often telling herself that her work was 'not good enough', that she wasn't 'exercising properly', that her hair 'wasn't right', etc. Through psycho education about communication styles and thinking traps, we employed strategies such as 'taking the thought to court' from CBT, and put our detective hats on to explore the evidence around Ellie's academic performance, exercise plans, morning routine, etc. All the evidence strongly indicated that she was a bright and hardworking student, well informed around healthy exercise, although perhaps doing a little too much sometimes, and had independently implemented a sensible morning routine, without much help and guidance.

Through careful and authentic reflections, I tried to highlight how incredibly well she had coped with the loss of her father, her best friend, two school moves and how she was taking care of herself and her mother. These reflections were captured on one of the paper sheets we always had on the table during our sessions, and I asked Ellie to add to them in her own words as and when she felt comfortable to do so. By the sixth session, Ellie needed no prompting to write them down and added her own reflections as well. We then developed a series of compassionate affirmations that Ellie could use when she noticed the 'not good enough' thoughts. Gradually, these reflections and affirmations told Ellie's story in a more positive and compassionate light, as she found strengths, successes and positive personal qualities in her experiences.

TOP TIP

People with self-critical thoughts can often find compassion-focused support a helpful first step in therapy, to recognise and reduce critical self-talk, often leading to improved self-perception and self-esteem over time.

We also used imagery to look at Ellie's body in terms of where she felt emotion, what she enjoyed about her body and what her hopes were for herself in the future. Ellie talked about wanting a family one day and how she worried that she might not be able to have children as her periods were becoming irregular. Using OARS from MI, we explored what was maintaining Ellie's difficult relationship with food, which appeared to be most closely related to feeling in control rather than keeping a low weight. Through open questions, we explored the areas where Ellie felt she needed more control and what would help. OARS provided a framework to check understanding and also to say out loud some of the issues that Ellie had felt she needed to keep silent about for fear of upsetting her mother. For example, with few rules and boundaries at home, Ellie could feel unsupported and uncontained.

Over the weeks, Ellie's mother had joined us for the last 5–10 minutes of each session, during which time Ellie and I shared some pre-agreed feedback about our discussions. Ellie's mother had also asked for some further information and guidance, so I had provided some leaflets and psychoeducation resources around communication and self-esteem, which she also struggled with. With this working relationship already in place, Ellie and I developed a plan with her mother around having more routine and structure at home, including around food and exercise, to support Ellie further. Ellie also developed a personal change plan with a view to valuing the function of her body over form, promoting her overall health and recognising she was worthwhile of time, support and care.

Towards the end of our work, Ellie reported that our approach had helped her view herself and her body in a more compassionate and less critical light, which helped develop her psychological and physical health. This included reaching a healthier BMI. In summary, a holistic approach to managing risk and working with underlying causes rather than 'symptoms' enabled a psychological focus to our work and brought about physical and psychological change, thus reducing overall risk.

Maisie: Creative artwork formulation and self-narration (20 sessions)

Maisie was in her 30s when she was re-referred to a community mental health team, following her third and traumatic mental health section and inpatient hospital stay. Briefly, Maisie had a long history of emotional distress as a result of multiple experiences of abuse and had recently lost her mother. Maisie had also reported dissociative depersonalisation at times, although 'zoning out' was more common at the start of our work. A maintaining stressor was that Maisie was working in the family business with two relatives with whom she had a challenging relationship (Figure 14.4).

Prioritising the therapeutic relationship and drawing upon Maisie's identified strengths and difficulties, a timeline that Maisie could populate was initially developed as the template for the formulation. Maisie explained that she preferred to draw and scribble rather than talk about some 'issues', which informed our collaborative style from the outset. The use of art within psychotherapy has been well documented (e.g. Greenwooda, Leachbe, Lucockcf, & Nobled, 2007; Huss & Sarid, 2014), and Karaca and Eren (2014) provide a persuasive argument for the use of creative artwork in case formulation. They describe how creative artwork can facilitate further understanding around thoughts, emotions and behaviour as well as the client's perception of themselves and others (Conrad, Hunter, & Krieshok, 2011). A full case report of Maisie's therapeutic journey based within the relevant theoretical literature was recently published (Parry & Lloyd, 2017).

In summary, we developed a picture and symbol-based timeline of events, thoughts and feelings as a preliminary framework for formulation, with a view to developing a full story and shared understanding. The progress of the timeline, accompanied by open explorative questions and reflections, facilitated a shared understanding of Maisie's past and how she related to it, as well as understanding how certain events still affected her now. The process also meant that the assessment and formulation aspects of our work were collaborative from the beginning, with a shared spoken formulation emerging.

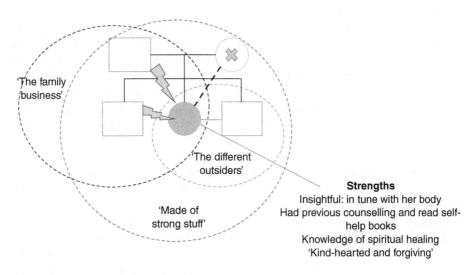

Figure 14.4 Genogram with added aspects of the formulation

TOP TIP

'Bear witness to the evolving story with its nuances of meaning, characters, emotional patterns, consistency, and uncharted courses' (Metzger, 1992, p. 71). People who have experienced certain traumas may have gaps or unintegrated parts of their life story. Being present as the story is told, reconsidered and even re-storied through an accessible medium can be a powerful therapeutic process. 'We think an important determinant of the response to trauma is the narrative strategies deployed to story trauma, including those used by professionals and scholars' (Weine & Chae, 2008).

By our fourth session, Maisie said she had added most aspects to the timeline and reflected that she was ready to 'do something with it'. When I asked what she meant, Maisie said she was ready to 'do the therapy'. I asked Maisie what she hoped for through the therapeutic process and she identified three goals: 'feeling more herself, feeling more present, and feeling more confident'. Drawing on SFBT approaches, such as scaling and coping questions, and using some of the information Maisie had shared with me about reading self-help books and spirituality resources, I explored how far Maisie had come already and the resources she had employed. Keen to maintain our collaborative approach, I explicitly linked some therapeutic options to experiences and exercises we could try and asked Maisie what she would like to try. The result was to use the following series of activities interchangeably and, with OARS, to facilitate change and maintain the focus:

- Mindful meditation and colour breathing.
- Exploring how Maisie was interpreting her butterfly spirituality cards in terms of her own qualities and resources.
- Practising a body scan exercise as another grounding technique.
- Using strengths-based approaches from positive psychology to explore how her strengths and talents were supporting her recovery, particularly in relation to curiosity, information gathering and problem solving.
- Maisie had been a keen painter before her most recent hospital stay and began painting again. She would bring her paintings to show me, which were often based on what she was learning about herself through our sessions. The paintings offered another platform for reflective discussions around healing and self-worth.
- Maisie would share traumatic experiences from her past during our sessions, usually during or after a particular exercise. OARS were sensitively employed to check meaning and summarise how she was developing a more cohesive interpretation and narrative around traumatic experiences.

As our sessions came to a close, I explained what a privilege it had been to work with her and that my usual practice was to write a Goodbye letter (from CAT) to summarise salient points from the process. Maisie said she would do the same and that we would swap them in our last session. I was keen for Maisie to hear the tone of my letter, so I read it aloud to her in our final session before giving it to her. I reflected upon her motivation, resourcefulness, strength of spirit and open mind, all of which had led to some significant changes in a relatively short space of time. Maisie's 'Goodbye letter' was in the form of a painting, which she told me about in some detail in relation to elements of our work together. Due largely to Maisie's creativity, this was one of the more integrative and fluid pieces of therapeutic work I have undertaken; it illustrated the power of a client's motivation for meaningful change.

TOP TIP

One of the many privileges of our work is that we can learn from incredibly strong and resilient people. Working with Maisie highlighted this honour very explicitly for me, which made me reflect on how I capture these learnings. A consequence ever since is that I keep an anonymised written record of what I learn and from whom, so I can continue to grow personally and professionally through my work. It can be difficult to make time for additional note-keeping in a busy schedule, although it can be an invaluable process!

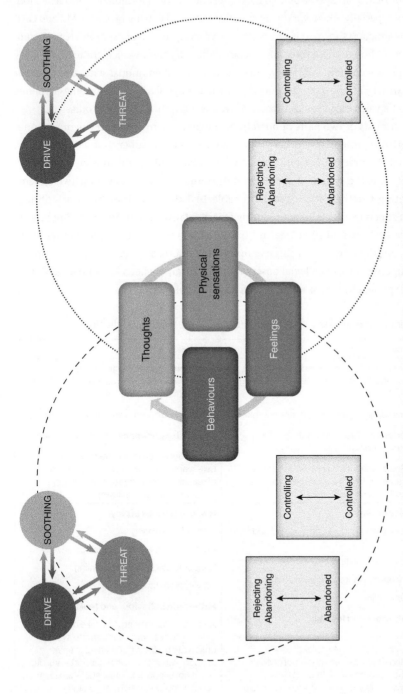

Figure 14.5 Formulation structure for considering individual and systemic parallel/contrasting pressures and influences

INTEGRATIVE TEAM FORMULATION

Integrative approaches can also be used to good effect for personal formulation and reflection, and staff teams, especially when working in complex settings. Drawing on CBT, CMT and CAT, I developed the structure shown in Figure 14.5 some years ago for supervision and team formulation purposes. Although these three approaches all have a cognitive element to them, CMT also brings explicit recognition of how we operate in different emotional states and how our physiology is wired to respond to stressors in particular ways. CAT also contributes dynamic considerations between ourselves and others, as well as our relationship with ourselves.

The model consists of two parts or operational circles, one to represent the practitioner and the other to represent the 'other', who may be a client, supervisor, colleague, etc. The idea is that the practitioner can explore what is happening within their system in a brief period of time, the system of the other in the same time, and how these two systems may be operating together. The example in Table 14.1 describes how I as a practitioner experienced a supervisory relationship during a particularly difficult restructuring process within an organisation, and what I learnt from the supervisor when I explored their operational circle. For the purposes of this example, we will look at a six-week period, during which time supervision and collegial observations have largely been suspended, and both parties were experiencing stress at individual and systemic levels.

Table 14.1 Mirroring processes in practice and supervision in a team under stress

Practitioner (me)	Supervisor
Thoughts: I am not wanted, not valued, not seen as a priority, not supported; what if something goes wrong and I am blamed?	**Thoughts**: I am not wanted, seen as a redundancy option, not supported, can't make a single mistake
Feelings: Stressed, upset, annoyed, frustrated, anxious	**Feelings**: Stressed, upset, annoyed, anxious
Physical experiences: Tiredness, tension, sleep disruption, recurring colds	**Physical experiences**: Tiredness, tension
Behaviours: Social withdrawal at work, less active in team settings, reduction in reflexive practice and creativity, missed work on days due to illness	**Behaviours**: Social withdrawal at work, risk-averse decision-making, tightening of relational processes (e.g. supervision, observations, case reviews)
Reciprocal roles in play:	**Reciprocal roles in play:**
Perception of being criticised ↔ critical of self and others	Isolated ↔ isolating
Alone/isolated ↔ and isolating	Unrecognised ↔ unrecognising
Unseen and unheard ↔ distancing from others	Unappreciated ↔ unappreciating
Unwanted ↔ unwanting	Unwanted ↔ unwanting
Patterns in behaviour and feeling:	**Patterns in behaviour and feeling:**
Engage less with supervisor – feel less support – become more anxious – engage less with colleagues – feel more isolated – feel more anxious – 'not good enough' thoughts – feel criticised through lack of engagement and feedback – overwork to compensate in terms of therapeutic contacts and note keeping	Anxious about making a mistake or being criticised by seniors – withdraw to avoid observation – feels threatening to seek support – struggle to offer support – anxious about not supporting junior staff – anxious about being criticised by other staff – increased isolation and anxiety

Practitioner (me)	Supervisor
Impact on the tripartite emotional regulation system:	**Impact on the tripartite emotional regulation system:**
THREAT: System in operation most of the time in work, stifles reflexivity, solution finding, connection seeking and creativity	**THREAT**: Overly active – affects working relationships, professional identify and wellbeing
DRIVE: Strive harder in some areas to compensate for losses in other areas	**DRIVE**: Focus on paperwork and record-keeping to prove competence and value to organisation, rather than relationships
SOOTHE: Difficult to engage at work and at home, due to tiredness and stress	**SOOTHE**: Difficult to engage at work and at home
Outcome: Imbalance in emotional regulation system affecting overall wellbeing, productivity and sense of self at work	**Outcome**: Imbalance in emotional regulation system affecting overall wellbeing, productivity and sense of self at work

In summary, although the pressures upon both parties were somewhat different, the outcomes were similar. Working through this model of reflection and awareness, albeit in a rather piecemeal and less cohesive fashion than that illustrated in Table 14.1, enabled us both to have some difficult conversations and explore how to reconstruct our supervisory relationship, offering each other more support and owning our less helpful coping strategies.

> Compassion isn't about letting yourself or anyone else, for that matter, off the hook. It involves compassionately seeing ourselves & others in the context of tricky lives, tricky influences & tricky biology. We say goodbye to blame & hello to responsibility. (Dr Mary Welford @DrMaryWelford)

TOP TIP

A key learning for me as a practitioner from Compassion-Focused Therapy is that self-care and self-kindness often require taking more personal responsibility for difficulties, requiring further action (and less avoidance) than I am sometimes comfortable with. However, this approach has reshaped how I work with challenges and difficulties, as well as giving me the permission to say 'no' rather than taking on too much, providing a compassionate, non-threatening framework for difficult conversations, as outlined in the example. Compassion can be tricky to fully embrace for ourselves but it can make a big difference!

MEMORY RETRAINING WITH COMPASSION

Typically, in the UK, memory-retraining courses for people with progressive memory difficulties are based on memory training tasks and CBT approaches for memory-related mood change. However, after running several such courses (usually over four sessions),

I became increasingly aware of two common difficulties that seemed to affect many of the older people accessing the service that were not being addressed through the training:

1. Self-criticism and frustration, which further impacted upon short-term memory function.
2. Fear of the future without reflecting on past and present strengths, qualities and abilities.

In response, people who came for a memory assessment and identified as being self-critical and fearful were offered an adapted pilot course, in place of the usual provision, which followed the structure shown in Table 14.2 (each session lasted two hours). The course included the usual memory training tasks and CBT approaches, but also involved CMT approaches, mindfulness tasks and an adapted exercise from narrative therapy.

Table 14.2 Session plan for a four-week memory training programme

Week One	• Psychoeducation around memory and influences that affect memory • Recognition and recall quiz • Introduction to mindfulness for memory, with a brief presentation on the scientific evidence behind mindfulness for cognitive function
Week Two	• Compassionate imagery task • Practical planning exercises around memory retraining (e.g. associations, mind maps, imagery related to words and processes). Homework: to undertake a related exercise at home • Introducing CBT techniques to reduce memory-related distress (e.g. common thinking traps, challenging negative automatic thoughts, activity diary – summary 'checking questions' below) • Soothing body scan exercise
Week Three	• Compassionate self-talk task and visualisation • Recap and group discussion following homework in relation to practical planning exercises around memory retraining from week two (what worked, didn't work, what will each member try next?) • Recap of CBT techniques and group discussion (what worked, didn't work, what will each member try next?) • Soothing body scan exercise
Week Four	• Recognition and recall quiz (results checked against scores in week one) • Adapted tree of life exercise (Dulwich Centre: https://dulwichcentre.com.au/the-tree-of-life) and group discussion and strengths and abilities the group can carry forwards • Group feedback and goodbye

RECOMMENDED QUESTIONS FOR GROUP MEMBERS BETWEEN SESSIONS WHEN HAVING TROUBLING THOUGHTS OR WORRIES

1. Is the thought logical?
2. Where is the evidence for the thought/belief?
3. Is the belief realistic?
4. Where is the evidence against the thought/belief?

5. Would your friends/family/colleagues agree with the thought/belief? What might they say?
6. What would your closest friend say about your thought/belief if you told them? What's the *kind way* to think about this?
7. Does EVERYONE share your thought/belief? If not, why not?
8. Will the thought/belief seem bad in one month, three months, six months or one year's time?
9. Might you be fortune-telling with little evidence that the worst-case scenario will actually happen?
10. What makes the thought/belief so terrible, awful and horrible? If a friend came to you with the same thought/belief, what would you say to them?
11. What do you know about yourself to cope with this difficulty? Who can you talk to about this?

The outcomes of this more integrative approach were very encouraging, with similar results across three pilot groups. Consequently, this short course became a standard alternative to the eight-week memory-retraining course for people who struggled with self-criticism and frustration around their memory difficulties. Although we were pleased to see the anticipated outcomes from these groups, there were some delightfully unexpected outcomes too. Some of the anticipated and realised outcomes were:

- Scores on the memory quizzes improved from week one to week four.
- Adding the mindfulness exercises provided another practical task for the group to do together and discuss, which strengthened relationships in the group.
- The psychoeducation around memory, mindfulness, mood and cognitive function was well received, with group members reporting that they felt more confident and in control with additional information about their condition and what could help, rooted in the evidence base.
- Considering the evidence base for the approaches employed to help memory function led to group members being more hopeful for maintaining their cognitive abilities and motivated to do the exercises.
- The addition of mindfulness and compassionate self-talk exercises raised group members' awareness of their critical self-talk and ability to develop a compassionate alternative.

There were also some pleasant surprises:

- Group members began to use emotional language and shared personal experiences with each other much more quickly than in the standard groups.
- Group members made recommendations to each other (peer-led learning) based on their experiential learning in between the group sessions. Unlike some of the standard treatment groups, all members always undertook some homework tasks and readily volunteered information back to the group. In essence, there was a greater sense of shared experience.

- The Tree of Life task from narrative therapy was introduced to offer a framework within which to focus on positive qualities, characteristics, precious gifts from others, skills and abilities. The exercise also brings together elements of a person's story over their lifetime. Many group members would not only discuss the process at length in the last session but let us know after the group had ended how they had shared their tree with family and friends, reflecting on how much they had to love and life for, rather than focusing on loss.
- Across the groups, members continued to meet in the hospital café after their group sessions had completed, not wishing to lose their new support base.

TOP TIP

Group therapeutic spaces can be wonderful places for all sorts of therapeutic relationships to flourish, with the right balance of engaged facilitation and group member autonomy.

Integrating therapies in an appropriate style suitable for both client and therapist can be a challenge. One helpful framework can be to consider a structure for therapy that can facilitate the weaving and navigating that often take place in a therapeutic encounter. The following '10 Rs' structure may be helpful to bear in mind for trainee therapists and will alter depending upon the nature of therapy with each client.

Before the session:

1. **Re-orientate** – check over notes and review any homework given.
2. **Recharge** – get in the right frame of mind for that client to meet their needs.

During the session:

3. **Re-acquaint** – welcome the client and help put them at ease.
4. **Re-establish the relationship** – a lot can happen in between sessions, so attend to the relational needs to re-establish safety and trust.

Pre-session/early-session talk – light smalltalk offers a chance for you to observe how your client might be feeling:

5. **Recap** – check with your client whether they would like to say a quick summary of the session, or whether they would like you to. Alternatively, both parties can state something they thought was important. Try to end on a positive or hopeful note.
6. **Revision** – agree on a relevant homework task to cement or consolidate something in the session.
7. **Re-schedule** – make a suitable appointment/confirm date and time for the next session.

After the session:

8. **Re-formulate** – at the end of the session or after the session, consider your formulation and update as necessary.
9. **Revise** – according to the nature of the session and any amendments made to your formulation, revise the approach/intervention/goals you have planned.
10. **Reflect** – critically appraise how the session went in terms of the therapeutic relationship, your conduct and the overall aims of the intervention and client's needs. Take to supervision.

─────────────── DISCUSSION QUESTIONS ───────────────

1. What may be some of the service-level barriers to offering an integrative therapy programme to a client?
2. What therapist attributes or characteristics may prevent a therapist offering an integrative therapy programme?
3. How do biases in the literature base influence the provision of integrative therapies across statutory services?
4. What may be some of the benefits to working with an integrative style?

─────────────── KEY TERMS ───────────────

Integrative psychotherapy (therapy or counselling; transtheoretical therapy) A combined approach to therapeutic work, which involves designing a personalised course of therapy for a client, taking into account their needs. Integrative therapists work on the assumption that no one therapeutic approach is a good fit for everyone, so they bring together aspects of different approaches based on their theoretical knowledge and the client's formulation. Approaches that share commonalities, such as person-centred therapy (PCT) and Solution-Focused Therapy (SFBT), can be brought together, although so can approaches that operate within contrasting frameworks, such as Motivational Interviewing (MI) and Cognitive Behavioural Therapy (CBT).

Integrative therapies Some therapeutic approaches have evolved and developed to encompass different strands from a variety of modalities. For example, Cognitive Analytic Therapy (CAT) (Chapter 8) draws on cognitive and psychoanalytic approaches, focusing on thoughts, feelings and behaviours, as well as relational patterns with ourselves and others. Similarly, originally stemming from Relational Frame Theory (Matoff & Booth, 2018), Acceptance and Commitment Therapy (ACT) has been described as a spiritually integrated approach (Santiago & Gall, 2016), also combining elements of cognitive and behavioural theories and introducing what are often known as 'third-wave' therapeutic techniques, such as diffusion and mindfulness. Relatively modern integrative approaches to therapy are becoming increasingly popular and evidence-based, as discussed in previous chapters.

Integrative perspective A flexible and inclusive approach to utilising a variety of therapeutic modalities (Greben, 2004), as illustrated in Figure 14.1.

─────────────────────────── FURTHER READING ───────────────────────────

- *International Journal of Integrative Psychotherapy* – an established and useful resource for peer-reviewed empirical studies, reviews, case studies and position papers.
- O'Brien, M. (2007). *Integrative Therapy: A Practitioner's Guide* (2nd ed.). London: Sage.
- Center for Integrative Psychology – web resources available at: www.brainoptimiza-tionmi.com/therapy-west-bloomfield-mi-faq/web-resources.html

REFERENCES

Berry, K. & Danquah, A. (2016). Attachment-informed therapy for adults: Towards a unifying perspective on practice. *Psychology and Psychotherapy: Theory, Research and Practice, 89*(1), 15–32.

Bowlby, J. (1969/1982). *Attachment and loss: Vol. 1. Attachment.* New York: Basic Books.

Castonguay, L. G., Eubanks, C. F., Goldfried, M. R., Muran, J. C., & Lutz, W. (2015). Research on psychotherapy integration: Building on the past, looking to the future. *Psychotherapy Research, 25*(3), 365–382.

Conrad, S. M., Hunter, H. L., & Krieshok, T. S. (2011). An exploration of the formal elements in adolescents' drawings: General screening for socio-emotional concerns. *The Arts in Psychotherapy, 38*(5), 340–349. doi: 10.1016/j.aip.2011.09.006

Greben, D. H. (2004). Integrative dimensions of psychotherapy training. *Canadian Journal of Psychiatry/Revue canadienne de psychiatrie, 49*(4), 238–248.

Greenwooda, H., Leachbe, C., Lucockcf, M., & Nobled, R. (2007). The process of long-term art therapy: A case study combining artwork and clinical outcome. *Psychotherapy Research, 17*(5), 588–599. doi: 10.1080/10503300701227550

Holmes, J. (2001). *The search for the secure base: Attachment theory and psychotherapy.* London and Philadelphia, PA: Brunner/Routledge.

Hughes, R. (2016). *Time-limited art psychotherapy: Developments in theory and practice.* London: Routledge.

Huss, E. & Sarid, O. (2014). Visually transforming artwork and guided imagery as a way to reduce work-related stress: A quantitative pilot study. *The Arts in Psychotherapy, 41*(4), 409–412. doi:10.1016/j.aip.2014.07.004

Karaca, S. & Eren, N. (2014). The use of creative art as a strategy for case formulation in psychotherapy: A case study. *Journal of Clinical Art Therapy, 2*(1), 1–8.

Kozarić-Kovačić, D. (2008). Psychopharmacotherapy of posttraumatic stress disorder. *Croatian Medical Journal, 49*(4), 459–475.

Lambert, M. J. (1992). Psychotherapy outcome research: Implications for integrative and eclectic therapists. In J. C. Norcross & M. R. Goldfried (Eds.), *Handbook of psychotherapy integration* (pp. 94–129). New York: Basic Books.

Matoff, M. & Booth, R. B. (2018). Circumstances to integrate acceptance and commitment therapy with short-term psychodynamic psychotherapies. *Cogent Psychology, 5*(1). doi: 10.1080/23311908.2018.1453595

McLean, H. R., Bailey, H. N., & Lumley, M. N. (2014). The secure base script associated with early maladaptive schemas related to attachment. *Psychology and Psychotherapy*, *87*(4), 425–446.

Metzger, D. (1992). *Writing for your life: A guide and companion to the inner worlds*. New York: HarperCollins.

Modic, K. U. & Žvelc, G. (2015). Helpful aspects of the therapeutic relationship in integrative psychotherapy. *International Journal of Integrative Psychotherapy*, *6*, 1–25.

Parry, S. & Simpson, J. (2016). How do adult survivors of childhood sexual abuse experience formally delivered talking therapy? A systematic review. *Journal of Child Sexual Abuse*, *25*(7), 793–812.

Parry, S. L. & Lloyd, M. (2017). Towards reconnecting: Creative formulation and understanding dissociation. *Mental Health Review Journal*, *22*(1), 28–39.

Quraishi, M. (2009). CAT effectiveness: A summary. *Reformulation*, *32*, 36–38. Available at: www.acat.me.uk/reformulation.php?issue_id=5&article_id=85

Rubino, G., Barker, C., Roth, T., & Fearon, P. (2000). Therapist empathy and depth of interpretation in response to potential alliance ruptures: The role of therapist and patient attachment styles. *Psychotherapy Research: Journal of the Society for Psychotherapy Research*, *10*(4), 408–420. doi: 10.1093/ptr/10.4.408

Santiago, P. N. & Gall, T. L. (2016). Acceptance and commitment therapy as a spiritually integrated psychotherapy. *Counseling and Values*, *61*(2), 239–254.

Tasca, G. A., Sylvestre, J., Balfour, L., Chyurlia, L., Evans, J., Fortin-Langelier, B., Francis, K., Gandhi, J., Huehn, L., Hunsley, J., Joyce, A. S., Kinley, J., Koszycki, D., Leszcz, M., Lybanon-Daigle, V., Mercer, D., Ogrodniczuk, J. S., Presniak, M., Ravitz, P., Ritchie, K., Talbot, J., & Wilson, B. (2015). What clinicians want: Findings from a psychotherapy practice research network survey. *Psychotherapy*, *52*(1), 1–11.

Weine, S. M. & Chae, S. (2008). Trauma, disputed knowledge, and storying resilience. *Paper presented at Trauma: Development and Peacebuilding Conference, hosted by International Conflict Research Institute (INCORE) and International Development Research Centre (IDRC)*. Available at: www.incore.ulst.ac.uk/pdfs/IDRCweine.pdf

Westra, H. A. & Norouzian, N. (2018). Using motivational interviewing to manage process markers of ambivalence and resistance in cognitive behavioral therapy. *Cognitive Therapy and Research*, *42*(2), 193–203.

Zarbo, C., Tasca, G. A., Cattafi, F., & Compare, A. (2016). Integrative psychotherapy works. *Frontiers in Psychology*, *6*. doi: 10.3389/fpsyg.2015.02021

COMPARATIVE SUMMARY TABLE

Therapeutic Modality	Approach	Style	Aims	Desired outcomes
Psychoeducation	Varies from a leaflet or online course to in-session explanations to courses delivered by experts or peers.	Collaborative approach preferred and expert position to be avoided but depends on the therapeutic stance. Sharing knowledge, skills and experiences.	Facilitating understanding and skills for client and/or their network to enhance wellbeing.	A new understanding of self, a new narrative. Insight and empowerment. In some approaches, adherence to a particular intervention/wellbeing.
Brief CBT	Direct, empirically based, formulation-driven. Delivery face-to-face or can incorporate elements of internet, telephone, Skype, individual or group.	Collaborative. Therapist provides direction in use of core CBT interventions. Client completes homework using self-help resources.	Negotiated realistic goals from the start. Aim is to achieve maximum benefits from limited sessions focusing on identified treatment priorities.	Reduction of symptoms, improved mood, functioning and wellbeing. Monitored via repeated psychometric questionnaires, subjective self-report and objective progress towards goals.
Motivational Interviewing	Direct, empirically based, goal-driven. Involves a shared understanding of the client's frame of reference, rather than an explicit formulation. Usually face-to-face with individuals (sometime telephone or Skype).	Collaborative, non-expert model, building on elements of PCT but with more guidance from the therapist. Key techniques are used to structure conversations in therapy to move towards the client's identified goals.	Promote informed choices, autonomy, empowerment and movement towards the client's chosen goals for enhanced wellbeing in alignment with their personal values.	Improved cohesion between values and actions, enhanced wellbeing and healthy choices observed and actioned through addressing target behaviours.
Time-Limited Person Centred Therapy	Following client agenda, centred on needs of client and relationship, use of non-verbal content, flexible structure. Number of sessions negotiated.	Non-directive, empathetic, acceptance, genuineness, focus on therapeutic relationship and depth of client emotive and embodied experience, client/therapist equality.	Expansion of self-awareness, uncovering potential/personal values and personal meanings, integration of parts of self, convergence of real/ideal self.	Qualitative evaluation of the therapeutic relationship, shift in perception of self and relationships. Reduction in symptoms indicating lack of self-acceptance.
Brief Family Therapy	The approach is direct and flexible. The number of sessions offered is approximately 10. Main techniques are: reframing and paradoxical interventions.	The therapist's style is directive and strategic. The relationship is collaborative and the therapist assumes a 'not knowing' stance.	To change the family's maladaptive patterns of communication. To assist the family in adopting more successful solutions to problems.	Reduction of problems noticed by the family and corroborated through a follow-up telephone communication.

Therapeutic Modality	Approach	Style	Aims	Desired outcomes
Solution-Focused Brief Therapy	The approach is guiding and flexible, with the therapist taking a facilitative role. Key components are: solutions talk, scaling, future-focused questions and imagery. The number of sessions should generally be as few as possible.	The therapist's style is curious and conversational. The relationship is collaborative, and the therapist assumes a 'not knowing' stance, exploring exceptions, strengths and change.	To encourage positive change and confidence by broadening and building on 'exceptions' and minor positive changes to initiate and establish a positive spiral of continuing change.	Increased attention to the positive and the future; a positive sense of self, ability and autonomy to initiate and maintain change for greater wellbeing.
Short Acceptance and Commitment Therapy	Direct. 1 session – 24 sessions. Flexible delivery.	Collaborative, psychoeducational, experiential and use of metaphor and analogy. Non-expert position: we are in the same boat.	Increased psychological flexibility and valued living. Goals agreed in therapy that relate to Values. Client is responsible for making meaningful therapeutic change.	Measured/monitored via process and outcome measures. Who notices change client and therapist observe changes. Review sessions negotiated at the beginning.
Brief Dynamic Interpersonal Therapy (DIT)	Psychodynamic, semi-structured, short-term, one-to-one therapy (16 sessions).	Combines core elements of the analytic stance with a more active, engaging and collaborative style.	To connect presenting symptoms of depression with a core, unconscious, repetitive pattern of relating. To enhance client's mentalisation capacity. To promote security in the attachment system. To relieve depression and enhance wellbeing.	To relieve symptoms of depression and anxiety. To enhance interpersonal functioning. To improve capacity to understand mental states of self and others. Diagnostic tools such as PHQ-9 and GAD-7 are frequently used to measure the efficacy of DIT in symptom reduction.
Psychodynamic Interpersonal Therapy (PIT)	Individual therapy.	Collaborative and negotiating in promoting meaning and understanding.	Facilitating greater relational awareness and understanding of feelings.	Developed understanding of personal styles of relating and the management of feelings.
Cognitive Analytic Therapy	Individual and group therapy and used in personal and professional development sessions. Also used with teams and organisations in contextual/consulting formats.	A shared collaboration and emotionally engaging activity of making meaning.	To develop greater relational awareness through recognition, reformulation and revision in promoting change.	Improving awareness and understanding of personal relational styles.

Therapeutic Modality	Approach	Style	Aims	Desired outcomes
Internet-delivered CBT	Indirect, flexible, tailored delivery. 24-hour availability allows for utilisation as per user's preferred schedule. Offline support from trained professional available.	Service is user-centred. Based on core CBT principles delivered online through mixed multimedia content (videos, interactive tools, text, exercises).	Similar to face-to-face therapy, achievable after an 8-week use of the online content and feedback from supporter.	Reduction of symptomatology noticed by user, measured by validated questionnaires and corroborated through follow-up with healthcare professional.
Brief Forms of Art Therapy	Provided in the form of one-to-one therapy and group work. Delivered by art therapists (art psychotherapists) who have trained at Master's level.	Art therapy is influenced by a range of psychotherapeutic approaches so the style varies greatly, e.g. psychoanalysis, psychodynamic psychotherapy, CBT, Cognitive Analytic Therapy, Systemic Therapy, Solution-Focused Brief Therapy, person-centred therapy. Client-focused collaborative approach to understanding the meanings of the artwork is preferred.	Facilitating the client to use art-making as a language to express thoughts, ideas and feelings that they find difficult to put into words. Assisting them to explore the meanings in their artwork and develop their insights. Encouraging the client to explore their creativity as a resource for their health and wellbeing.	The client gains an enhanced sense of their own resources and feels empowered in their recovery process. The experience of verbal and non-verbal communication in the therapeutic relationship helps them to better communicate their feelings in other relationships in their lives.
Brief Uses of Compassionate Mind Training	Usually (not always) direct, no fixed number of sessions, flexible delivery, appropriate for service/systemic interventions.	Collaborative, predominantly a coaching model of learning new skills and applying them within compassionate framework.	Develop understanding of own brain; redress balance of the three systems; develop compassionate mind to bring to difficulties; reduce shame and self-criticism.	Behavioural change but also change in relationship with self, tone of self-talk, and more able to be kind and compassionate to self and accept the same from others.
Brief Interventions in Hospital Settings	Both direct and indirect. Emphasis on team working and flexibility of approach as opposed to protocol-driven work.	Discusses balance between collaborative and directive approaches, given different situations, taking into account issues of power and facilitating change.	Aims to improve physical and emotional wellbeing through supporting coping, adjustment or management of health needs.	Discusses difficulties in direct measurement and highlights value of other mechanisms of evaluation, e.g. attendance rates.

INDEX

Page numbers in **bold** indicate tables and in *italic* indicate figures.

self-criticism *see* Compassion Focused
   Therapy (CFT)
self-harm, 115–18, *117*
self-psychology, 100
SFBT *see* Solution-Focused Brief Therapy
   (SFBT)
shame
  psychoeducation, 193, 196
  see also Compassion Focused Therapy (CFT)
Shapiro, F., 191
Shimazu, K., 191
short-term family therapy, 53, 65–77, **220**
  assessment, 71
  attempted solutions, 69, 72, 76–7
  case study, 76–7
  circular causality, 68
  course of therapy, 70–5
  cybernetics, 67–8
  evaluation, 75–6
  evidence base, 70
  follow-up interview, 75
  goal setting, 69, 72–3
  homeostatic mechanisms, 67, 69
  interventions, 69, 70, 73–5, 76
  observation teams, 70, 71
  paradoxical interventions, 74–5, 76
  practical guide, 70–5
  reframing, 73–4
  restraining technique, 74–5
  Strategic Approach, 68–70
  systems theory, 66–7
  termination, 75
  theoretical foundations, 66–8
  theoretical model, 68–70
  therapeutic relationship, 70
  therapist's stance, 70
Silverstone, L., 145
SMART goals, 7, 10, 11, 56, 86
Snyder, C. R., 62
social anxiety
  Acceptance and Commitment Therapy
   (ACT), 90–1
  Brief Cognitive Behaviour Therapy
   (BCBT), 13–15, *14*
social constructionism, 54, 193
socioeconomic status, health outcomes
  and, 159
Solomon, G., 142
Solution-Focused Brief Therapy (SFBT), 28,
  52–62, **221**
  art therapy, 144, *144*
  assessment, 53, 56
  basic tenets, 54–5
  case studies, 59–62
  compliments and encouragement, 59
  coping questions, 59, 62

course of therapy, 56–7
evaluation, 57
evidence base, 54
goal setting, 56
groups, 61–2
homework, 57, 62
hospital settings, 167
interventions, 57
miracle question, 42, 57–8, 60,
   61, 62, 71, 144
practical guide, 56–9
psychoeducation in, 61, 62
scaling questions, 58–9, 60, 61, 62, 144
techniques, 57–9
termination, 54, 57
theoretical introduction, 53–4
therapeutic relationship, 56, 59
somatic conditions, internet-delivered CBT
  (iCBT), 175
soothing rhythm breathing, 131
soothing system, *126*, 127, 130
Springham, N., 137, 140, 142, 146
stepped-care approach, 191–2
Strategic Family Therapy *see* Mental
  Research Institute (MRI) model of
  Strategic Family Therapy
stress control, 192
Strosahl, K., 84
student counselling service, 24
suicide prevention, 117
Sullivan, H. S., 100, 102
summaries, in motivational interviewing,
  39–41, **40**, 44, *44*, 46, 47, *47*, *48*
support systems/networks, 189
symbolic behaviour, 99
symbolisation process, in psychoeducation, 193
Systemic Family Therapy, 53
  see also Mental Research Institute (MRI)
   model of Strategic Family Therapy
systems theory, 66–7
Szapocznik, J., 65, 70

Taft, J., 23
Target, M., 102
team formulation, 211–13, **212–13**, *212*
theoretical models, **xix**
therapeutic relationship, xiv–xv, *xvi*
  art therapy, 138, 150
  Dynamic Interpersonal Therapy (DIT),
   105, 106, 107, 109
  integrative approaches, 205–6, *206*, *207*
  motivational interviewing (MI), 37, 38–9, **41**
  psychoanalysis, 99–100
  short-term family therapy, 70
  Solution-Focused Brief Therapy (SFBT),
   56, 59